Keep It Up, Harry Potbelly!

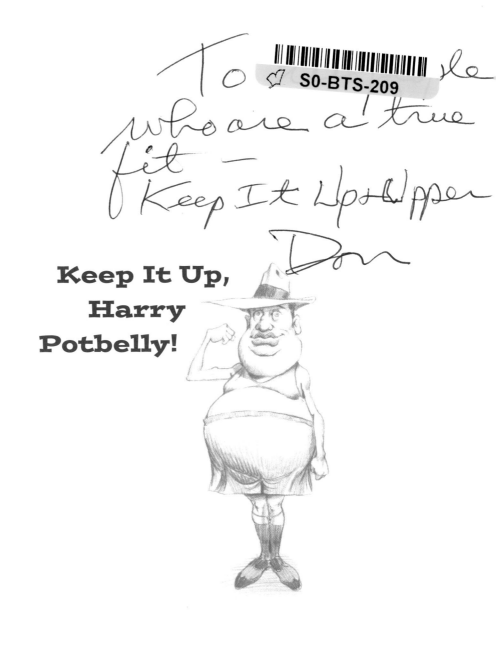

S0-BTS-209

Keep It Up, Harry Potbelly!

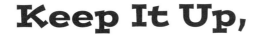

A Doctor's Lighthearted Guide to Robust Health

by **Don Linker**, M.D., M.P.H.
with Edwin Heaven

Illustrations by Steve Haefele

Feel Better Press

Keep It Up, Harry Potbelly!
By Don Linker with Edwin Heaven

Illustrations by Steve Haefele

Published by:
Feel Better Press
28 Lyford Drive
Tiburon, California 94920
dlinkerd@aol.com

Publisher's Cataloging-in-Publication
(Provided by Quality Books, Inc.)

Linker, Don.
     Keep it up, Harry Potbelly! : a doctor's lighthearted
guide to robust health / by Don Linker with Edwin Heaven
; illustrations by Steve Haefele. – 1st ed.
     p. cm.
     LCCN 2005921758
     ISBN 0-9765745-0-0

     1. Health. 2. Exercise. 3. Nutrition. 4. Physical
fitness.   I. Heaven, Edwin. II. Haefele, Steve.
III. Title.

RA776.L56 2005   613

Table of Contents

Exercise

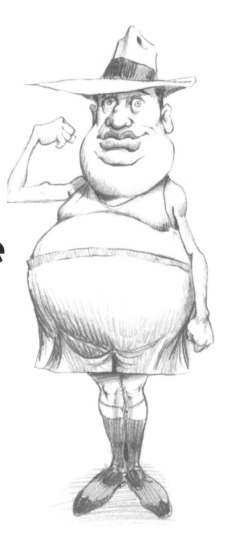

WARNING!

This book contains irony and other trace minerals.

Introduction

A Doctor's Digit

Health and fitness are no laughing matters. Not until now, that is. This book will make your gut giggle (laughing, not lifting) while giving you a doctor's inside information on how to get healthy and stay healthy. Dr. Linker makes it easier by pointing out the don't-miss nuggets of information in gray boxes. As a urologist, he knows how to get to the point.

To lift your spirits while you lift your weights and read this motivational stuff, you will be accompanied on your journey to health by a rotund private eye named Harry Potbelly, his blonde bombshell client, Monica Marinara, and by the Three Ripped Pigs. While learning all about diet, strength, and cardio exercise, you will meet Theresa Triathlon and Rip Van Ripple, the personal trainer, and you will laugh your way through "pecs and peccadillos" and "dumbbells for dummies." On your agenda are saunas and steam baths, saturated fat, spinach, sweet potatoes, and the stinking rose—everything

Strange-But-True

Your first strange-but-true fact, unknown in the Western world until now, is that three balding men in white lab coats came up with the theory that regular physical activity and a diet rich in fruits, veggies, whole grains, and plenty of rest may help prolong life. These experts developed their theory while on the back nine somewhere in Minnesota, and they failed to mention that this regimen prolongs life for only about half a year.

When they published their report, Dr. Driver, Dr. Woods, and Dr. Putts left out this part: no matter how hard you work out, how good your diet and how much rest you get, a healthy life gives you about 182 days more of breathing in and out. ⟝

Working out. Oh, not that! Eating well. And breathing! Mustn't forget to breathe. Very important, breathing. The mechanics of breathing are broken down into two parts:

1. IN

2. OUT

In... out... in... out...

While practicing this exercise, avoid, at all times, asphyxiation, strangulation, drowning, being buried alive, and sleazy motels lacking air conditioning.

you wanted to know about losing weight and getting fit while having a good time.

Some of us will make it to the ninth hole; some of us will get as far as the eighteenth green. And, some of us won't make it to the fourteenth tee. As they yelled, "Fore!" those three doctors figured out that it's all fore-ordained. Call it genetics, call it fate, call it doom. Call it dumb. There are just so many years available in that evanescent,

slowly deteriorating body of yours. That's right, the natural order of things dictates that you will live x number of years.

Your years may be dramatically shortened, by smoking cigarettes or smoking crack, driving under the influence or driving without a seatbelt, or by taking a bullet for dear old Uncle Sam. Even if you are lucky enough to dodge the bullet, your body has software programmed to go so far, and no farther—except for that half year you might get if you work out, eat right, and breathe.

Sooo, why break a sweat? Why strain yourself on the Stairmaster to stay trim? Why eat low-fat, low-carb, low-sugar, high-protein food?

Why bother? The Doc recommends that you better bother because a healthy person feels better, works better, plays better, and maybe makes love better. You will even think better, and people will think better of you.

With this book, you will give yourself an additional six months (maybe more, for good behavior), and your breathing time will be all the more enjoyable. Unless, like Dr. Putts, you are lost in a sand trap somewhere in Minnesota, sinking down, down, down.[1]

A mere lad of 22 in 1937, Jack LaLanne was into bodybuilding. In those days, instead of climbing onto a machine to max out your deltoids, your abs, and your pecs,

---

[1]Leave it to Dr. Putts to find quicksand in Minnesota. If you find yourself in the same situation, puppy-paddle like heck while screaming, "Help, HELLLP!" at the top of your lungs, unless they are filled with sand. Then, recite the 23rd Psalm: The Lord is My Shepherd... he maketh me to lie down in... glub glub...

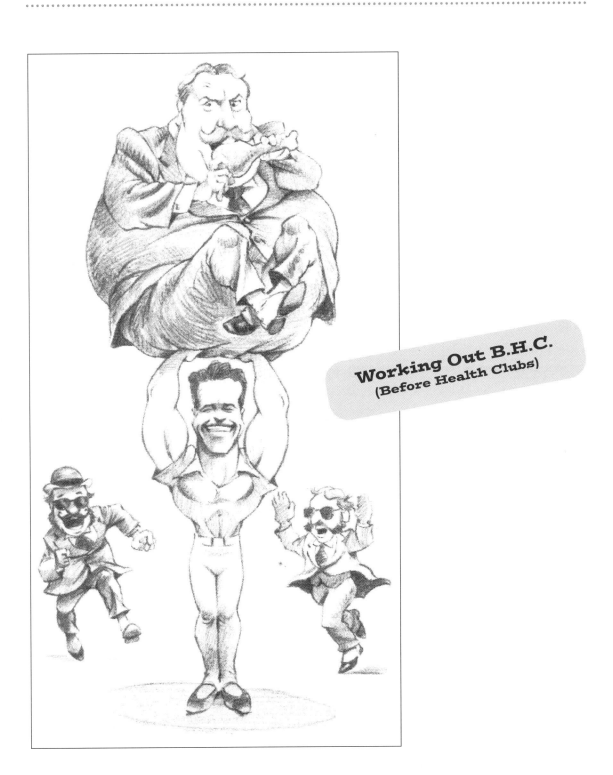

Working Out B.H.C.
(Before Health Clubs)

you lifted large, ponderous objects. Jack made himself famous when he lifted a brand new Model A Ford filled with voluptuous young belles who were dressed in tight corsets and petticoats and dancing barefoot to a bawdy rendition of "Charlotte the Harlot."

Some say that one of Jack's friends was inspired by the belles to invent the dumbbell. Some say the word dumbbell originates from the practice of removing clappers from bells, thus rendering them soundless (dumb).

After the Model A stunt, Jack lifted William Howard Taft, a large, ponderous Republican, high off the ground. Always a publicity hog, Jack had planned to curl the curly-mustachioed 27th President of the United States twenty-seven times. But, old Tubby Taft screamed so loud, and his secret service gorillas pummeled Jack so hard, that he was unable to curl the prez more than thirteen times. Yet, it's a record that stands today—although the young bodybuilder had trouble standing for several weeks.

As this book went to press, Jack was still standing at 89 years old. Why is he so healthy? He works out like crazy. And, he purees raw vegetables and fruits together in a blender and tosses it down, every day. And he has a secret.

See if you can guess what it is:

a. He is careful to avoid the harmful rays of the sun.

b. He sleeps in a coffin.

c. He drinks large quantities of blood.

d. All of the above.

If you chose D, you win. Jack LaLanne is a vampire!

Your First Workout

Half of the people who buy books and start exercise programs or diets quit within two months. The main reason is that damn Chapter One. Sooo, to hell with Chapter One!

Chapter Ones are the ones that tell you the tedious, hypothetical, complicated stuff you are supposed to do before you can begin to do what it is you really need to do. (Lawyers and accountants probably write these chapters.) The stuff like body mass, heart rate, blood pressure, sphincter control (think I'm kidding? check out a hatha yoga manual), cholesterol level, and body fat index.

When you read everything in Chapter One that you are supposed to do to get your butt off the couch, the deeper you plant your butt and the sooner you fall into a deep ZZZzzzz…

Before going to Chapter Two, let's take a Pop Quiz (unless you are too pooped).

You are reading this book because:

- Your TV is broken and you have nothing to read?

- You have the musculature of Gumby?

- Your idea of health food is Raisinets?

HINT… ....

Want to get off the couch? Try this:

1. Put feet on the ground (practice using a slow, concentrated movement).

2. Slowly stand up (for even better results, avoid stepping on your pet).

Or skip this and go on to Chapter Two.

- Your doctor nixed your request for anabolic steroids and prescribed this book instead?

- You have not had a good laugh (or a decent job) since the Clinton Administration?

- Passing the time reading this sure beats passing a kidney stone?

- You are stuck on a stationary bike to hell?

- Oprah Winfrey recommended this book?

- Oprah Winfrey did not recommend this book?

- You really, truly want to look like a million bucks?

Whatever your reasons for picking up a funny book about working out and dieting, you are already on your way to a healthier, sweatier, longer, more relaxed and fun life. Keep it up!

A Sorely Needed Sit-Up

A Hard-boiled Tale to Help You Get Rid of that Soft-boiled Belly

Harry is a private investigator, or, as they say in pulp fiction, a gumshoe, a shamus, a private eye. Very clever, that Allan Pinkerton[1], who turned the "i" in investigator into an "eye," thus coining the term, private eye. The first P.I. in the United States, Pinkerton used a giant eye for his logo; his motto was, "We Never Sleep." Perhaps this was because he did not eat enough turkey: more turkey = more tryptophan = more sleep.

Monica Marinara, the ravishing wife of Muscles Marinara, showed up in Harry's office one morning. She wanted to hire him to find out if her brawny hubby deserved an "M" branded, permanently, into his forehead. The tantalizingly top-heavy Monica

Turkey Talk

Do you get sleepy after eating a big turkey dinner? Dr. Andrew Weil, author of the book, *Spontaneous Healing*, writes, "L-tryptophan, an amino acid and a natural sedative, is a normal constituent of turkey flesh and it is also the starting material from which the brain makes serotonin, which calms you down and makes you sleepy."

Since L-tryptophan works best on an empty stomach, Harry will be better off eating a piece of leftover turkey at bedtime, rather than a whole Thanksgiving dinner. —

---

[1] The son of a Glasgow policeman in Scotland, Allan Pinkerton emigrated to the United States in 1842 and became a deputy sheriff in Chicago. In 1852 he formed an elite group of detectives who solved railway robberies, and he also served as chief of Union intelligence in the Civil War. No couch potato, Pinkerton pursued criminals across state lines. He died at age 65 and might have lived another six months if he had drunk less Scotch, eaten more vegetables and walked instead of riding in railroad cars.

More Turkey Talk

Dr. Weil also says, "While we're talking turkey, I'd suggest getting an organic one for your Thanksgiving table. Most commercial turkeys contain growth hormones, antibiotics, and other additives incongruous with a healthy body. After a delicious dinner, take a good long walk and breathe. " ⎯

Donut Holes

Somebody ought to tell him that the best thing about a donut is the hole. It takes an hour of brisk walking to burn off just one Krispy Kreme. Get this: the calories in a single KK donut range from 200 for a glazed to 390 for a glazed devil's food old-fashioned.

Would you walk 2 to 4 miles for a Krispy Kreme? ⎯

said to Harry, "I think the muscle-bound monkey is cheating on me."

Monica had almost as many curves as the Grand Prix. If she were a car, Harry thought, she would be a fire-engine red Ferrari, and taking a peek under her hood crossed his mind. He also wondered why a husband in his right mind would take a detour when he had such a classy chassis at the finish line?

His mouth full of Krispy Kreme, Harry garbled, "Whychoo shushpectim?"

"I didn't quite catch that," Monica said, absent-mindedly flicking away sugar glaze that had landed on her glossy, golden tresses.

Chewing and swallowing before he could speak, Harry stared gratefully at the way her tomato-red tank top molded itself, like a Wonder Woman costume, to her lavishly displayed cleavage. "What lungs!" Harry thought. "Must be a great swimmer."

Monica was a bottled-blond version of the raven-haired stunner who portrayed Wonder Woman on TV. What was her name? Something Carter. Amy Carter? No. Oh yeah, Lynda Carter.

Harry repeated the question, "Why do you suspect him?"

"Because he's been staying out late every night for the past three weeks, that's why," Monica said. "And when I ask him where he's been, he tells me the same baloney—some 24-hour gym for naughtiness."

Naughtiness? "Oh, he probably said Nautilus," Harry said, making a mental note to check out the Nautilus health clubs. And, it certainly will not hurt Harry to get familiar with a health club; he may be a flatfoot, but he's not a flat-belly. In fact, everything about Harry is round, including that prodigious paunch.

Leaving Harry a retainer, Wonderbra Woman sashayed out of his office. Harry dashed out and cashed the check

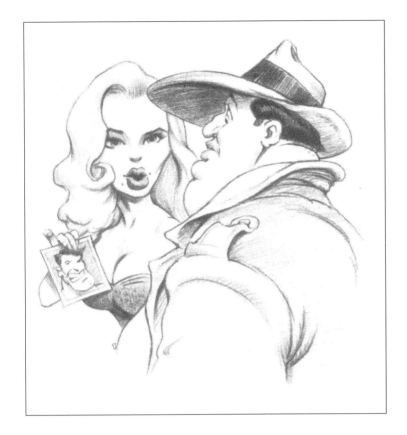

Get a Move On!

Little does Harry know that swimming benefits the upper body, midsection and legs all at once. It also improves cardiovascular fitness with little or no stress on the joints. No need to fret about torn ligaments and sore knees: swimming is the most ergonomic cardio workout of all. ⟶

while the ink was still wet, then stopped off at the local cholesterol emporium to quickly stock up on his old pals, Bud and Sara Lee. Health food? Forget about it. Harry's idea of health food is a cough drop, and his idea of fresh produce is Juicy Fruit gum.

Setting off in his vintage DeSoto to find the menacing meathead, Muscles, the alleged adulterer, Harry found him right where Monica said he would be, at the local health food cafe. Harry parked his car and taped an "Out of Order" sign to the parking meter, a little trick of the trade (a trick that

doesn't work for Harry, who currently owes $436 in parking tickets, just about enough for a year's membership at a health club).

Stepping into a pizza parlor to grab a huge, greasy, gooey slice of pepperoni pizza to tide him over, Harry came out just in time to spy Muscles leaving the cafe. Huffing and puffing after him, Harry ruminated on how he hated to walk. His motto is, "Why walk when you can drive?"

With thighs the size of tree trunks and a barrel chest, Muscles moved so fast that Harry struggled to keep up. "This guy is in

Walking Wisdom...

Three hours of walking a week may reduce your chances of getting prostate hyperplasia, a condition that can give you a prostate the size of Rhode Island. The larger the prostate, the slower the urine flow; so, don't get pissy, get walking. ◀

tip-top physical shape, hale and hardy," Harry said to himself. "I wish he were more like the Hardy in Laurel and Hardy."

Dressed in a snug, mud-brown, single-breasted, three-button suit—with two buttons missing and the third about to burst—Harry looked large in the barge and loose in the caboose.

Where Muscles' taut stomach can be called a six-pack, Harry's is a keg. Muscles' rippled abs resemble a washboard, while Harry's resemble an old Maytag washer loaded with goose down pillows. Muscles has killer abs. The closest Harry ever came

Fashion Advice...

Men, don't publicize your fat, conceal it. Wear single-breasted suits with padded shoulders and pleated side vents to hide your rubber tire. Full-figured women, steer clear of anything clingy and avoid wearing red and white striped muumuus—you may be mistaken for a circus tent. ◀

to killer abs was when he collared a killer named Abbie; "Killer Abbs" they called him.

In great shape, Muscles is what they call "ripped," while Harry will be what you might call R.I.P.'d (yeah, six feet under) if he doesn't lay off the pizza.

Like that famous bespectacled kid wizard, Harry Potter, Harry has a scar on his forehead, which is probably the reason he wears that old fedora. He got the scar when he leaned into a motel window to snap incriminating photos of a client's spouse in a compromising position (which as a rule meant that Harry could compromise a higher fee, from both spouses). Suddenly, the subject of the photos looked up and slammed the window shut, slamming the camera into Harry's frontal lobe, causing a gash (ouch) and costing him cash (double ouch). The camera left a temporary Nikon imprint and a scar, not in the shape of a lightning bolt, but big, fat, and shaped like a giant burrito, one of Harry's favorite snacks.

Although Harry is fond of burritos, the lard-infused, bean-filled tortillas are not fond of him. Not only do they enlarge his XXL size beanbag, they give the flabby flatfoot flatulence (go ahead, say flabbyflatfootflatulence fast, three times). He may tail a cheating spouse or two, but when the spouse gets wind of Harry's wind, the chase is over.

That's one rumbling rump Harry's got, a pair of booming buttocks. Not only does he suffer from excessive wind, he is also easily winded from being so flabby and out of shape. He can hardly keep up with the slow-

Exercise...

Instead of resting in peace (or pizza), Harry needs moderate exercise and a low-fat, high-fiber diet to reduce his risk of colon cancer and heart-threatening hypertension. Exercise unclogs arteries by raising HDL (good) cholesterol and lowering LDL (bad) cholesterol. —

Gone With The Wind

Harry doesn't know that, unlike the movie, *Gone With the Wind*, with proper diet and exercise, and an adequate supply of activated charcoal capsules or Bean-o, acidophilus, and enzyme supplements, the wind is gone. Here's another tip for keeping your friends: soak beans in water for several hours, pour off the water, then cook with fresh water. A low-cost, low-fat source of protein, beans are good for you! —

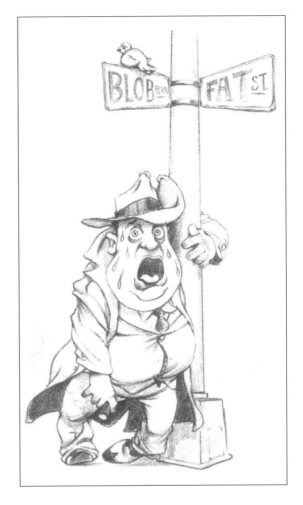

est guy on the street, let alone someone as energetic as Muscles Marinara.

There he is, our pal Harry, shuffling along, puffing loudly, sweating profusely, his fleshy face flushed and bloated, his ponderous footfalls growing heavier with each step—ker-thud! ker-thump!

You know you're out of shape when you can't make it across the street during the green light, and a few flights of stairs make you feel like you're climbing the Empire State Building in cement shoes. The view at the top may be breathtaking to some, but to Harry, who pants like a chubby Pekinese, it literally takes his breath away—he carries an inhaler, for his asthma. Uh-oh, today he forgot it, which is why he wheezes and pants, nearly falling flat on his full and reddened face.

With Harry gasping behind him, Muscles stopped at a newsstand to buy a bodybuilding magazine called *Muscular Madness*, giving Harry a chance to catch his breath and peruse his favorite monthly, *Mammoth Mammaries*. The covers of both magazines featured topless and well-built, greased-up bodies, except that Harry's cover girl had a body that looked as if it had been handled by more than one Beverly Hills surgeon.

While Harry peeked at the chesty models, his old friend, Doctor Linker, walked up and said, "Hey, Harry!"

"Hey, Doc," said Harry. "I see you got rid of that little paunch of yours."

"I've been working out. Maybe you should try it."

Harry slapped his gut and wisecracked, "Great bellies are made, not born."

To which the Doc retorted, "So are clogged arteries."

Harry's whole face frowned, a rotund face, balloon-like and ruddy from years of hard knocks and harder liquor. With all those frown lines, it looked like a pink volleyball.

"Get to the point, Doc," said Harry. "A guy can stand only so much advice."

"My point is, the greater the waist, the greater the risk."

"Risk? Ha! I eat risk for breakfast!"

"Yeah," the Doc said, "probably the sugar-coated kind." Giving Harry's arm a squeeze, he said, "Look at you, you're soft as bacon fat. That's a pudgy predicament you've gotten yourself into. To get out of it, I have three little words for you: diet, strength, and cardio."

"You will excuse me if I don't write them down—I'm working," said Harry.

"Better you should work out," said the Doc. "The cardiovascular kind, to burn calories, strengthen your heart and lungs, and lower your blood pressure. And, with the right diet…"

"Cease and desist," said Harry. "Lecture's over. Can't you see I'm on a job? Look over there. See that big ox reading the muscle mag? I'm shadowing him."

"So I noticed, Harry. I have a gut feeling he's noticed you have a shadow as big as Alfred Hitchcock's."

"Well, they don't call me Harry Potbelly for nothing."

"It wouldn't hurt to lose some of that pot. You know what they say about too much pot."

"Yeah," chortled Harry. "It causes the munchies."

"Which is exactly what you don't need! You know, Harry, you don't have to lose all of your excess weight. You don't even need to be thin. Even fat men who are fit have a lower death rate than thin men who are not fit."

To this, Harry replied, "I don't think I can stomach losing my stomach. Why would I want to lose my most notable feature? It's what I use to belly up to the bar."

Keeping a stealth eye glued to Marinara, he added, "I just hate this whole diet and exercise thing. It's so prissy, with everybody prancing around in tights and do-rags, acting like kung-fu masters. And those yoga freaks twisted like pretzels. Just the thought of it makes me woozy."

"All of that can make you healthy, Harry. "Heart disease, obesity, and diabetes are so high in our society because physical activity is so low, and people are eating waaay too much, far too often. I remember when people used to lug their own golf clubs, push lawn mowers, get a little workout, break a little sweat. Remember?"

Harry nodded as the Doc went on, "Now they drive around in electric golf carts and on those 15-horse-power, ride-on mowers with more gears than a Harley. People have simply stopped walking, except to get to their cars! And, parking lots even have shuttle buses so you don't have to walk a block or two to get to your car. I know a guy who, every day, spends a half-hour on the Stairmaster, and when he goes to the office, instead of climbing the stairs, he takes the elevator!"

"You may be right about folks being lazy nowadays," muttered Harry. "I happen to like elevators, and, I wish this mug I'm shadowing would take one once in a while. He's walking me ragged."

"Maybe you ought to drag that ragged sack of potatoes of yours to a gym once in a while, Harry. In fact, you are welcome as my guest, anytime."

"Nah! Remember how I hated gym in school? They called it Phys Ed, then. I wrote my own excuses, forging my mom's signature: 'Please excuse little Harry from Phys Ed. He's got athlete's foot...'"

Fat and Fit?!

According to the Cooper Institute for Research in Texas, you don't have to lose weight to be healthy, you just have to move. People who exercise, no matter what their weight, have a lower death rate than those who sit around. Increasing your life span could be as simple as walking thirty minutes a day. You can be fit and fat! —

Obesity

A growing overweight and obesity epidemic is threatening the health of millions of Americans in the United States, according to the Centers for Disease Control and Prevention. This is due to the growth of the fast food and snack food industries, an increasingly automated workplace, hours of daily television watching, and the replacement of walking with automobile travel for all but the shortest distances. —

More Facts on Walking

As much as he hates walking, Harry won't get hurt doing it. Walking has a low injury rate, and it strengthens the bones and the muscles. The average person burns 275 calories an hour walking a 20-minute mile; if you can walk the mile in 12 minutes, you burn about 585 calories an hour. And, lucky for Harry, the heavier you are, the faster you burn 'em: studies show that a 110-pound person burns about half as many calories as a 215-pound person walking at the same pace for the same distance. ⟶

"When were you ever 'Little Harry'?" asked the Doc, and they both laughed. "What will it take to get you to throw away those phony excuses?"

"You can't pay me to go to a gym."

"What if I told you that at my gym, the benches and machines are filled with attractive women?"

"Women?" Although this aroused Harry's interest, he noticed that Muscles was walking down the street, and so he took off after him.

"See you around, Doc," he puffed.

Crawl, Walk, Run...Walk!

Fitness Without Throwing Fits

While Harry Potbelly slogs along at a tortoise's pace, let's stop and look back. No, not a few minutes—a lifetime! Back when you were just a tot. Maybe you don't remember; then again, maybe you have seen yourself in those old home movies—your funny little stutter steps, the drool and the double chin, which hopefully you don't have anymore!

The fact is, you don't need home movies to know that, before you walked, you crawled, or maybe rolled. (Or, like Elvis Presley as a tot, you shook, toddled 'n rolled.)

As you tried to stand erect like the Homo sapien that you are, you fell on your cute little bum. And, every time you fell on your diaper-cushioned tush, you got right back up again on those pudgy little wobbly legs and kept on trying. Up, down, kerplop! Up, down, kerplop! Up, down, kerplop!

Over and over and over until you finally took those very first, very tentative, wavering steps that had everyone cheering like you

were a Kentucky Derby winner, even though you staggered like the town drunk, and a bowlegged one at that.

From crawling to walking, one day you graduated to running. "Run, Dick. Run, Jane. Run, run, run."

Many of you who graduated to running have dropped out of the race, particularly those of you with bad backs, or gnarly knees, or aching Achilles tendons. Which is why there may be a sign flashing in your head: "Walk. Don't Run."

If you are crawling, see a doctor or a physical therapist. If you are walking, be sure to do it briskly. Unlike running, fast walking is fitness with less emphasis on the footness—and the backness—and the knee-ness.

Have a Nice Day of Reckoning

Everyone has a day of reckoning, the day when they decide to walk that walk. It might come for you when you notice that you no longer fit into your favorite jeans, or your favorite chair. Certain body parts are spreading, like cream cheese, or they are dropping, like the Dow Jones. Gravity is taking its toll...

Your Day of Reckoning may come while you are walking the dog. If the dog is walking you, or perhaps dragging you—especially unpardonable considering the size of your Pomeranian—it's time to pound the sidewalk and walk off some pounds.

Walking is for Everybody, and Every Body

You have two ages: your chronological age (the one on your driver's license) and your physiological age (the way your brain and body function). A 58-year-old can function like a 38-year-old and, of course, vice versa, if he or she does not stay fit (or, stinks in math). Each person ages at a different rate.

Fast walking may make you look better, and regular walking may keep your mind young, too. Studies show that people who walk regularly are less likely to have memory loss (the better to keep track of your birthdays).

Several studies indicate that taking gingko biloba may improve short-term memory. Other studies refute that; which ones, I don't recall. Now, if I can only remember where I put the bottle of gingko biloba! I am sure it will come to me as soon as I get back from my walk. Now, where did I put my shoes?

Forgetting is a good workout. I do it frequently. I often forget why I walked into a

Postmenopausal

A study published in the New England Journal of Medicine reports that a daily brisk walk is 'heart healthy' for post-menopausal women. Those women who walked at least 3 miles or more per hour for at least 2.5 hours a week for an average of 3.2 years, were substantially less likely than sedentary women to develop heart disease and stroke. And it's never too late! Sedentary women who became active in middle adulthood or later had a lower risk of coronary events than their counterparts who remained sedentary. —

room; then, I walk out and suddenly remember why. Then, I go back and, once again, forget. Try repeating this exercise eight to twelve times. If you still don't remember, see someone about your condition. And, hey, at least you got a good workout!

The cool things about fitness walking is that it doesn't cause a fit. It's easy—start small, with a ten- to twenty-minute walk. The idea is to keep moving. Even the elderly stay healthier and happier and live longer when they are active. "Young at heart" is just another way of saying, "Keep that heart and body of yours younger" (and you can even hum the tune).

HINT...

Here's how to walk that walk:

Focus on good posture. Think tall thoughts. Imagine yourself as Shaquille O'Neal or Elle McPherson—tall, tall, tall.

No slouching. Relax your shoulders, widen your chest, pull your abdominal muscles gently inward. Good!

Now, keep your head and your chin up. Your hands should be relaxed, sort of cupped. Swing your arms (and dosey-do), but don't pump them, sway them. The upswing and downswing should brush past your body from breastbone to hip bone, from hip bone to breastbone.

And your foot: it should land heel first, then roll through to your arch and to the ball of your foot, then to your toes; push off from your toes.

Complicated? Not really. Just hit the heel, roll to the ball, and push off on the toe. All the while, swing your arms and keep your back straight.

Now, move on down, move on down that road. And, don't forget to breathe! As the TV ads say, "Just do it!"

Walk Fit

You don't need a treadmill, you only need the outdoors. If it is raining or snowing, walk inside a mall. If Michael Jackson can do the Moon Walk, you can do the Mall Walk.

Wherever you walk, do it at a fast clip. Try walking with a Walkman to get into a rhythm; use a single earpiece so as not to miss oncoming vehicles, and observe traffic signals.

Why drive or take public transportation when you can walk? In a big city, you may even get to your destination sooner. During a New York rush hour, someone timed a walker against a bus and a subway, and the walker beat them both! (He probably would have beaten them by more if he hadn't been mugged along the way.)

You can walk almost anywhere and make the most of it. Walk home from the supermarket using your bagged groceries as weights (ask for double plastic bags). If lugging groceries interferes with swinging your arms, consider using a backpack—just take care not to scramble the eggs.

As you approach your destination, go all out and really quicken your pace. If there are stairs, walk briskly up them. If there is a hill to climb, climb it like the Little Engine That Could ("Yes, I can, yes, I can!").

Is walking athletic? Absolutely, especially if you have athlete's foot.

Is walking therapeutic? Positively. When you walk 10 miles a week, you are much less likely to develop stomach troubles. And, walkers suffer less from erectile dysfunction

The Mall Walk

Many shopping malls open their doors early for walkers. Your advantages are a controlled, comfortable climate; no traffic or auto fumes; mall security on duty; and restrooms and water nearby. And, some malls encourage walkers with walking clubs, discounts and health check-ups. And, you can window-shop at the same time! ←

than non-walkers. To avoid erectile dysfunction (ED), you should also avoid smoking and drinking heavily, not to mention avoiding a swim in shark-infested waters. Maybe ED can be avoided by walking rather than riding in a limousine...

Wear Running Shoes to Walk?

Running shoes are okay for walking. To be on the safe side, tie the laces together (after you take them off). That way, they won't run off. Running shoes are notorious for doing that. If your shoes have Velcro instead of laces, lock them away in a closet (again, not when they are on your feet).

With walking shoes, you don't have to worry about them running away, although sometimes they like to walk around in the kitchen, their tongues hanging out as they sniff around for food. Should that occur, pick them up and stash them in a drawer. Don't worry, walking shoes are not very bright (if they were, they would be running shoes).

If you keep your walking shoes in a drawer, beware: they are flirtatious little devils and, given the chance, will hit on the socks, particularly sexy pantyhose from Frederick's of Hollywood.

Talk That Walk

If you get bored walking, find somebody to walk with you, so you can walk and talk. If the conversation is boring, stop talking. If you are still bored, try skipping. Skipping is fun. Skip to the store. Skip to the bank. Skip to the loo, my darling (if you owe the tax collector, you better not skip town).

Other ways to fight boredom:

- Get a Walkman (notice it is not called Runman).

- Dress like Nancy Sinatra and sing, "These boots are made for walking."

- Put a nice, thick slice of salami in each shoe. If your feet are vegetarian, try a tofu dog. Walk around all day giggling to yourself. Everything will seem funny, and smell funny, too.[1]

---

[1]Try the salami—it works! While writing this, I took a brisk walk with slices of Hebrew National salami stuffed in my shoes. Now, while I sit here writing—and while my shoes are walking around with their tongues out looking for salami—I'm giggling because my cat is licking the balls of my feet. Now, he's sinking his teeth into— owwwwch!

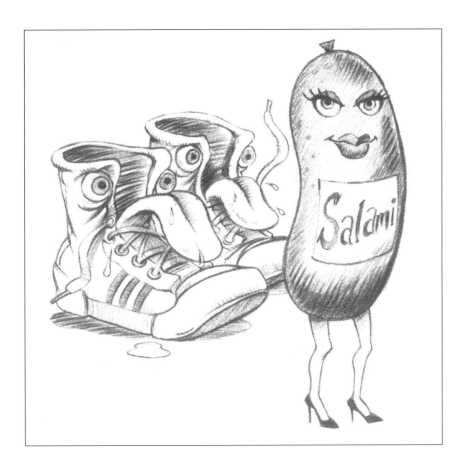

Walking Sticks

Walking may not be a trendy, overly hyped exercise program like Tai-Bo or Typo[2] or whatever it's called (Ty Cobb?). Although walking is not performed at an expensive health club using complicated machines, it is still an effective workout if you walk fast enough.

Research shows that some people find it easier to stick to a home-based fitness program, such as walking or push-ups (or shot-putting cats), because they can participate on a consistent basis. So go ahead, take a nice long walk (but watch out for potholes, Mr. Potbelly).

Walking regularly burns fat regularly. And, walking has a low injury rate compared to running (unless you fail to look both ways before crossing, or fall into an open manhole).

[2]Typo is very effective. It takes off weight by simply missing a letter or two. For example: fat becomes fa; or, 393 pounds becomes 93 pounds.

Walking is low-impact and easy on the hip bones, the backbones, the knee bones, and it's easy to talk and to listen and to smile while you walk.

Pregnant?

When you are expecting and you feel lethargic, go for a walk to get a surge of energy. Remember to walk tall, with your back straight. Don't hunch your shoulders: lead with your chest (and, as the months progress, you will have more of it to lead with).

Some women in their second trimester get the urge for pickles and ice cream. Go for it, as long as you walk, not drive, to get them. Or, drive to the store and walk the aisles at a brisk pace, as long as you are careful not to tilt the baby.

While carrying the little stranger, carry a water bottle wherever you go to avoid dehydra-tion. Rule of thumb: always drink before you become thirsty. After you feel parched, your delicate metabolism is already off balance.[3]

So, wash down your pickles and ice cream with lots of water, Mama.

Walking is Hip

Pushing a stroller? Take a stroll.

Over the hill? Walk up a hill.

Nobody walks more than homerun king, Barry Bonds; in fact, he holds the Major League record for walks. And, don't forget what Frankie Valle and the Four Seasons sang in that moldy oldie of theirs: "Walk like a man, fast as you can, walk like a man, my son."

---

[3]Avoid caffeinated beverages too, as they tend to cause dehydration. You can tell when you are dehydrated by checking your urine. Deep yellow color with an intense odor may mean that you need to drink more water (this test only works if you have not been eating asparagus, which can produce a strong smell).

A Sorely Needed Sit-Up

Part Two

The plot thickens, along with Harry's waistline... Here's Harry, right where we left him, perspiring, short of breath, bursting at the seams of his suit and hot on the trail of Muscles Marinara. Yes, bursting, because like a bloated bullfrog, Harry eats on the fly and the fry. If it's finger-lickin' good 'n greasy, Harry is in heartburn heaven. And if he keeps going the way he's going, he will slide into the hereafter way ahead of schedule.

Say "Cheese!" and Harry smiles. The cheesier, the bigger the smile. He needs to bypass all that cheese, before he needs a bypass.

Drumsticks

Instead of marching into the Colonel's place, Harry should be marching to the beat of a different drumstick (remember, dark meat has more fat; white meat is leaner 'n meaner). Instead of a Big Mac, he ought to have a big carrot. ⟶

Not only does he down a heck of a lot of donuts, hot dogs, and pizza, he drinks like a fish (and I'm not talking guppy, I'm talking gulpy—he gulps it down). Another name for Potbelly could be Beerbelly.

Right about now, he's so parched that it's time to fill'er up. This Marinara he's tailing is not stopping for anything. Muscles is on a mission. "A mission from hell," thinks Harry, who stumbles, then staggers, his pitiful lungs sending out a sickly gasp and his sizeable stomach releasing a loud rumble. Just as Harry expected, Muscles marches into a health club.

Figuring this is where Muscles plans to rendezvous with his alleged paramour, Harry lumbers in after him, to find that this isn't some textbook gym, or some religious-oriented shrine, or some nutritional spa, or even some all-day, all-night warehouse. It isn't a YMCA or a YWCA or a USDA, for that matter.

As he looks around at one of the oddest sights a gumshoe has ever laid peepers on,

Harry thinks, "Of all the gym joints in all the towns in all the world, he had to walk into Rick's Gym."

Rick's doesn't look at all like the gin joint in the movie *Casablanca*. It looks like Dante's *Inferno* to Harry and the sounds are just as hellish! Weird equipment whirring, bicycle wheels whirling, barbells banging, and all that heavy breathing. The puffing and panting and grunting sounds like a steamy porno movie.

Working out in a frenzy, guys are covered with tattoos from forehead to toe, adding to the carnival-of-pain atmosphere.

From bald eagles to Chinese dragons to leaping dolphins and flaming skulls, every one has inscribed his muscle bumps with permanent, personalized, bumper stickers.

"Is this the Marquis de Sade Gym?" wonders Harry. Some of the gnarly, grueling devices look straight out of a torture chamber from the Spanish Inquisition.[1] Talk about misery! To Harry, the place looked like a clammy nightmare in a Stephen King chiller.

The last time Harry stepped foot in a gym, his sizeable backside was snapped with towels until it was as pink as a

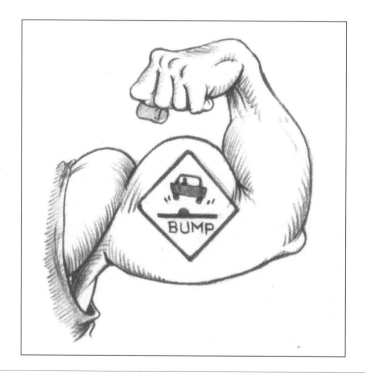

---

[1]In the early part of the 20th century in America, convicts were forced to climb onto rolling staircases to generate electrical power for prison facilities. It was cruel and unusual punishment, yet you should have seen the legs on these guys—quadriceps to die for! (Unfortunately, some of them did.)

baboon's. In high school when a gang of rowdy jocks, splashing and falling and guffawing around in the shower, caught sight of Harry's abundant flesh, they couldn't resist teasing and taunting him. They snapped his big behind with wet towels, until it was Harry that finally snapped and got into a fistfight.

He got suspended from school for a few days, while the rambunctious rowdies were out on their backs for a week. Once their casts and bandages were removed, they limped right past Harry whenever they saw him in the hallway, giving him a wide berth. Ever since that boyhood experience, Harry has harbored a strong dislike for gyms and jocks. And now, here he is in a gym surrounded by jocks—and also some good-looking Jills.

While keeping a furtive eye on Muscles, Harry glances around at all the dumbbells among the dumbbells, like the one trying to look cool while drenched in sweat. "Real drips," he thinks.

All the buffed guys are drips, their thick leather weightlifting belts tight around their waists, sweat pouring off their faces, their T-shirts dark and wet and

Potbelly Wisdom...

If you are too lazy to break a sweat, drops of sweat can be duplicated by splashing water all over yourself. Spring water works best. For the full effect, breathe heavily and try to smell real bad. ◄—

smelly... drips, all of them. Everywhere he looks, Harry sees sopping wet gloves clutching barbells, and soaked elbows pressed against the leather padding of the equipment. And, there is a mob of moistened muscles in Gore-Tex tank tops, Lycra shorts and all the rest of that trendy paraphernalia, peddling big bulky bikes that go nowhere fast, complete with flashing lights, and often with a personal TV set.

Some of the guys have shaved heads, burly shoulders, and big, beefy, bulging biceps like characters out of a Marvel comic book. In fact, their tattoos read like comic books.

Their pecs and lats and the hard-hammered musculature of their legs resemble exaggerated cartoons drawn by the likes of Stan Lee (creator of Spiderman), Bob Kane (creator of Batman), Shuster and Siegel (creators of Superman), or Johnson and Johnson (creators of dental floss).

"The only thing some of these characters need," Harry says to himself, "are masks and capes—Superjocks!—able to leap tall buildings in a single steroid injection."

Here at Rick's Gym, big flabby guts are few, especially a gut as colossal as Harry's. His big old potbelly is as much an endangered species as monogamy (or even the Monarch butterfly). And, speaking of butterflies (and clever segues), Harry is feeling some ol' butterflies deep inside that ol' potbelly, because he is admiring from afar a knockout with a face like Uma Thurman and the hard body of a triathlete. She's so hot, you could fry an egg

Wheatgrass

Wheatgrass is a green liquid extracted from sprouted grain, high in vitamins A, B, C, and E, as well as many amino acids. It may not substitute for 3 pounds of vegetables—it's more like a substitute for 3 pounds of lawn clippings—that is how it tastes. Proponents of the stuff claim that wheatgrass provides more pep than a cup of espresso. ▬

on her griddled (and thoroughly crunched) abs. She probably runs or bikes miles a day and every morning, bright and early, does the Australian crawl through frigid San Francisco Bay. And, Harry thinks, "She is probably just as frigid. The hotter they look, the colder they usually are. Her thermostat is probably stuck on subzero."

You know the type. She worships fitness. Instead of tequila shooters, she does double shots of wheatgrass.

This gal's idea of bliss is breaking the tape at the end of a 26-mile marathon. She probably has a heartbeat slower than the local Muni. If Harry ever got her alone in his office (he fantasizes), he would get it beating faster than a hummingbird on methamphetamines. Though considering his sad shape, to give a triathlon athlete that kind of workout would probably give Harry a coronary. (Talk about bad heart rates: Harry's is so obscene, it's rated R. Stick around. In a few more pages, I show you how to rate your heart.)

As Harry gawps, she turns around and gazes right back at him, and even throws in a big, pearly-white, sassy smile, along with a flirty wink (actually, it was just an eyelash that got in her eye). Now a bit smitten, Harry bashfully backs away, crushing a few hapless toes in the process. He darts a quick glance around to be sure he hasn't lost sight of Muscles Marinara, who is in the midst of his daily stretching routine.

Harry is beginning to notice that just about every face in this place has a goofy—no, make that euphoric, determined, and disciplined—grin on it; either they are smiling, cringing, or both. *The Agony and the Ecstasy?* The last time Harry observed this many happy campers, somebody had dropped a hallucinogenic substance into the water cooler at Camp Minnehaha.

Everywhere he looks, someone is beaming or some body is soaked to the skin and bursting with verve and vitality, even those little blue-haired old ladies in the aerobics rooms, gleaming with glee, their dentures sparkling. They are doing low-impact exercise to Barry Manilow's "Copacabana," but the way it looks to Harry, they should be

Bending Iron

To bend iron, the first thing a blacksmith does is heat it up. The same goes for pumping it. Warm up your muscles by starting every workout with an easy five minutes on a treadmill, rowing machine or exercise bicycle. ▬

Never Too Old

American Sports Data, Inc. reports that the 55-plus set is the fastest-growing segment of the fitness industry, with gym memberships increasing 378% in the past decade or so. Weight training not only slows the aging process, it can actually reverse it, with the oldest and weakest showing the greatest improvement. In a Tufts University study, a group of 90-year-olds improved their strength 174% after 8 weeks of weightlifting. Some studies show that strength training also encourages weight loss, lowers blood pressure, reduces the risk of diabetes, and produces favorable changes in cholesterol levels. ⎯

playing Wagner's "Gotterdammerung," or maybe "Taps."

Harry thinks the oldsters probably show up at the gym every day just to rub elbows with their perspiring peers. If he wanted to rub sweaty parts of the anatomy, he would go to a singles bar, instead of a gym.

He spies an elderly woman in a yoga position, snoring loudly, and someone else, hog-tied to a Pilates machine, hollering for help. Another silver-haired person is twisted and wrenched like a Bavarian pretzel. It's enough to make poor Harry break out in a rash.

A muscular Methuselah has a black toupee that looks as if it fell out of the blue onto his dome. The way his rug is whooshed up in the back of his head, the guy seems to be moving when he's standing still. The old fellow may be fit as a fiddle, but that toupee doesn't fit worth a pizzicato, and, what he lacks in hair on his head, he makes up for in his nose and ears.

On a flat utility bench lies an ancient artifact, drool dripping off his chin. Harry mutters to himself, "He could use one of those dental saliva-suckers, and a nurse to nudge him along so he can finish sleepwalking through his workout." Harry doubts that anyone over eighty can even exercise his pinky finger. In fact, he is the one in need of a nudging nurse. Just rolling out of bed in the morning is exhausting for P.I. Potbelly.

Harry is about to eat his words. In fact, he should eat words more often, since words contain zero calories, zero cholesterol, and zero fat. If he offends one of these elderly gents with big muscles, Harry might end up with a fat lip.

Bench Wisdom...

The correct way to do the bench press is to take a grip a little more than shoulder width, then lower the weight slowly, under control, to about the middle of the chest. Most important, begin the pressing motion from the chest itself while keeping your lower back pressed against the bench. Don't scratch your nose, or it might end up looking like Michael Jackson's. ⎯

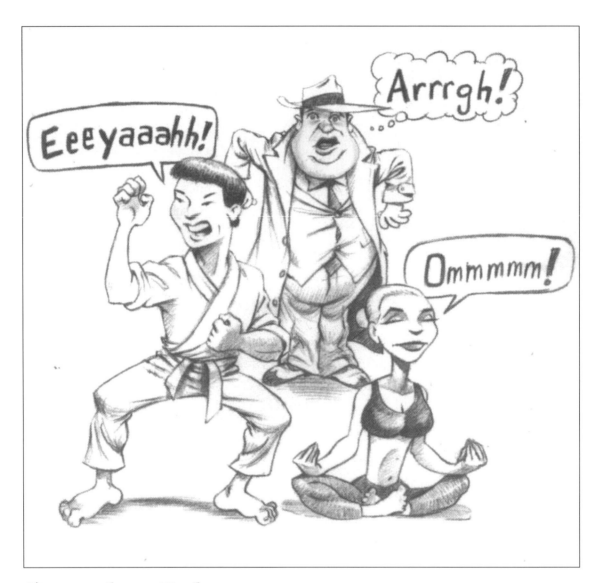

Strength vs. Endurance

Build strength with heavy weights and low repetitions. Build muscular endurance with light weights and high repetitions. Build me up, Buttercup, just don't let me down. —

The gent with the prodigious nasal hair begins to bench-press 120 pounds, his own body weight.

Harry grumbles a bit too audibly, and slinks away from the steely gaze of a 90-pound man in a wheelchair who is curling 20-pound weights.

HINT...

Some folks don't know diddly-squat about squats. Here is the correct way:

Squat down slowly while holding onto something for support (a walker is fine, or back up against a wall) and squat down only to where your knees are directly over your feet and thighs are parallel with the floor.

Any other technique will risk tearing knee cartilage (maybe even your shorts if you have grown a bit large in the barge like our Harry).

Did you know that people who squat are prone to arthritis of the knee?

Harry feels the glowering dagger stares of a stooped woman with a walker, who is doing limber little knee bends.

As Harry glances back to double check on Muscles Marinara, he notices the muscleman is surrounded by (what looks like) the Los Angeles Lakers Girls in skintight tops. The paunchy private eye wonders which one of these gaga goddesses is Marinara's mystery woman. He's also thinking, with a salacious smirk on his face, "Heck, this health gym isn't so bad after all!"

5 Sweat

The Good, the Bad, the Malodorous

It is now time to sweat like pigs; although, in fact, pigs don't sweat because they don't have sweat glands, which explains why they cool themselves off by wallowing in the muck.

Now, for a close look at sweat. Think of the sweat gland as a long, hollow tube resembling the Holland Tunnel during a traffic jam. Imagine ducts and pores lined up, bumper-to-bumper everywhere in the skin, and particularly in the armpits and the groin area.

As we all know, sweat stinks—or, does it? In fact, sweat has no odor. The unpleasant odor is the result of bacteria, which tends to collect under your arms on the hair follicles; the bacteria metabolizes proteins and fatty acids, creating a smell. Sweat glands are more abundant under your arms, which may be why deodorants and antiperspirants are applied only there, rather than to the entire body.

The average person has 2,600,000 sweat glands in his or her skin. You won't find them, thank goodness, on the lips, nipples, or external genital organs; and, for that, we should be grateful.

Mate Attraction

Scientists believe that the activity of the sweat glands helps to attract a mate (or, a checkmate, if playing chess causes you to sweat). ⟵

Why does skin taste salty after a workout?

Sweat has chlorine, chlorine attracts sodium, and together they produce salt in the body—sodium chloride, $NaCl$—which is important in regulating the pressure and flow of fluids between the blood and tissues of the body, and for normal nerve and muscle function. If you were a chef like Julia Child or Wolfgang Puck, you might say that sweat is too salty and needs Margaritaville.

How much do we sweat?

Vigorous activity can produce one liter of sweat an hour. If you live in a desert, it may be a lot more. If sweat were Cabernet Sauvignon, a liter would cost a pretty penny.

Can you name four great sweaters?

How about: Elvis, Satchmo, James Brown, Turtleneck.

What are some fun ways to work up a sweat?

(Aside from Olympian sex...)

How about cycle karaoke? That's riding an exercise bike while singing. You are literally spinning tunes, sweating so much the cyclist next to you feels like she is singing in the rain (when it pores, it rains).

The game of squash is another great, sweaty workout, and it goes nicely with turkey and cranberry sauce. The experienced squash player never takes his eye off the ball—otherwise, he might lose it (the eye, not the ball).

Long John Silver was a great squash player until he lost his eye; then, his leg got squashed and he lost that, too. He lost the Treasure Island map, he lost his parrot, his keys, and his ATM pin number. Ahoy me hearties! Squash is good for the heart! Long John lived a long life, and what was left of him was just a wooden peg, a tattered patch, and a pirate's laugh.

Ultimate Frisbee, now, that is really a fun workout. The game requires the speed and endurance of a soccer midfielder; the quickness and defensive savvy of a basketball point guard; and the hands of a football receiver. It is played on a 70- by 30-yard field and the goal is to advance the disc into an end zone with a series of passes upfield. Running while in possession of the Frisbee is a no-no, and so is catching it in your mouth (which not only eliminates a lot of drool but some of the world's finest four-legged players).

Each team fields seven two-legged players, and games can be 11 points or 3,267 points, depending on the amount of caffeine or Clif Bars consumed. Ultimate Frisbee may be the most aerobic sport, as players run between three and five miles at a sprint, during three or four games a day.

Basketball is another way of breaking a sweat, or if you are clumsy, breaking a leg. A little half-court game of one-on-one is okay, although with the head faking and popping long jump shots, not enough running may be involved. Two-on-two is better, because you can give 'n go, set up picks and screens, and even crash the board for rebounds. The best workout is full-court basketball, which requires running, jumping, and fast breaking, and—if you are good enough to play in the NBA—random drug testing.

Crooks tend to be healthy because they run a lot, mostly from the law. When caught, they get the third degree, which means they not only get a steady cardio workout but a heck of a third degree burn. If convicted, they get a lot of time to pump iron and take invigorating cold showers—great for the body!

Is there a cure for sweaty palms? Often an embarrassing condition, sweaty palms can be treated by medication and surgical procedures. Injection of Botox is one of the newest treatments. Cutting off the hands is the most effective.

Are steam baths and saunas beneficial? The body's core temperature usually rises one to two degrees while in the sauna, thus imitating a slight fever. You sweat buckets, which causes the cardiovascular system to get a workout, since the heart must pump harder and faster to move blood to the surface for heat exchange. Your heart rate may increase from an average of 72 beats per minute, on average, to 100 to 150 beats per minute.

Steams and saunas do offer the benefits of relaxation and the relief of muscle ten-

sion, as long as you are careful, since overheating may cause a heart attack, which is worse than heartburn.

A noted artist once told me that success is 1% inspiration and 99% perspiration, which explains why his art work is always so soggy. He was right—don't be a quitter. Keep on keeping on! And sweat your arse off.

By the way, there is no such thing as no sweat. It takes physical exertion to reach your health and fitness goals. Depending on your gender, it also takes a sturdy bra or jock strap (in the case of aerobics classes taught by a male teacher in drag, it may require both).

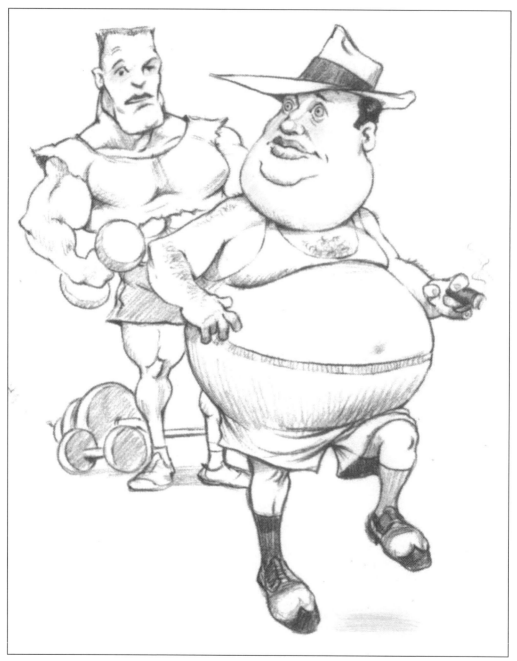

Rip Van Ripple

A Sorely Needed Sit-Up

Part Three
"Go ahead," said Dirty Harry, "make my delts!"[1]

A rippled-gut brute in a ripped-to-shreds sweatshirt, Rip Van Ripple poses a question to Harry: "Are you somebody's guest or are you here for a trial workout?"

Harry responds, "I am here for a trial, pal, and I plead innocent."

Picture this: a disgruntled Harry Potbelly in the men's locker room, stripped to his shopworn, threadbare boxer shorts, his prodigious gut soaking right through his grubby undershirt. He is sweating because he is grossly overweight, and because he is mortified.

The ripped guy named Rip has the puffed-up chest and inflated arms of the inveterate body builder, and one helluva reputation for helping people to lose fat and build muscles. In Harry's case, an easier task might be turning water into wine, or better yet, Gatorade. The unwieldy mass of flab standing there just might be Rip's greatest challenge.

Rip sees, at once, that Harry Van[2] Potbelly is a man who cultivates barriers and stumbling blocks. Take, for example, his footwear—street shoes, badly scuffed genuine alligator. Not wanting to discourage a potential client, Rip decides to let the shoes crawl by.

"Next time," Rip grins, "wear proper workout shoes."

"Yeah yeah, sure sure," says harried Harry. He's thinking, "There ain't gonna be a next time, pal. As soon as I get the goods, the bads, and the uglies on Muscles Marinara (over there squeezed among his hale and hearty harem), this place is history!"

He also thinks, "If this big palooka, Rip, doesn't wipe that stupid grin off his kisser, he will soon be munching on a saturated fat,

---

[1] That is deltoids, not Altoids. Delts are the three-headed muscle group of the shoulder divided into front, middle, and back; or, anterior, medial, and posterior. (You want svelte delts? See Part II: Strength.)

[2] Yes, a potbelly the width of a mid-size van.

knuckle sandwich, and I'll deliver it quicker than Domino's delivers pizza."

Rip gawks at the mousy brown fedora still perched on Harry's head. He says, "You gonna wear that thing?"

"Yeah, pal," Harry snaps, snapping the brim neatly, while giving Rip one of his patented, you-wanna-piece-of-me looks. "It's my, uh... sweat band."

Rip reluctantly leads Harry out of the locker room past a bunch of bodybuilders, their pumped-up pecs, quadriceps, and abs glistening with sweat.

Great Pecs

The pecs, or pectorals, are two groups of muscles that cover the chest. Great pecs can give a guy deeper cleavage than Pamela Anderson. And, great pecs can be uplifting news for women, too. (See page 53 for more on pecs.)

Quadriceps are the muscles on top of the legs, consisting of four muscle heads, some of which have beards. ⎯

Kiss that potbelly goodbye, Harry. Crunches strengthen lower, upper, and oblique abdominal muscles. Take care not to strain your back (later in the book, you will learn how to do crunches without crunching your back).

As Harry is led past the thick-skulled bodybuilders, he comes up with a few wise-cracks which he keeps to himself, such as, "Check out the big gluteus maximus on that guy. Look how he jiggles. The man needs to do a hundred push-ups in a push-up bra!"

Most people who like to work out rarely pay attention to others at the gym. They are too busy staying focused on what they need to do to stay healthy and fit, while staring at themselves in the mirrors. If the body-builders are thinking anything as Harry passes by, it is probably what a gallant sonofagun he is for putting his best foot forward (even if that foot is wearing endangered wildlife).

There may be one person in the gym who is a little wary of the roly-poly oddball working out in his drawers, street shoes, and fedora. And that person isn't Ralph Lauren, it's Muscles Marinara.[3]

We interrupt this chapter for a word from the author...

If you pick up this book because you thought it was an instructional manual for dummies, you may be wondering by now, "What the heck is going on here?"

1 Am I ever going to find out how to do a proper sit-up?

2 Or, learn the correct way to do an over-head extension?

3 Will I discover the secret to attaining buns of steel?

---

[3]Ralph Lauren has a clothing line called Polo. For the sake of Harry Potbellies everywhere, Ralph should come out with a chic line of clothing called Roly-Polo.

4 And, how to choose the right health club at the right price?

5 Will I pick up a few sure-fire pick-up lines?

6 Or, find out who put the ram in the rama-lama-ding-dong?

Here are the answers to your questions:

1 Yes

2 Yes

3 Yes

4 Yes

5 Yes

6 I dunno.

Health Clubs

Before choosing a health club, shop around. For example, guys look for girls, and girls look for guys. In some cases, guys look for guys, and girls look for girls. And everybody is looking for a good deal. Some fitness clubs do everything they can to entice you and to lock you into a purportedly low monthly price. Their hard sells for hard bodies may be sound business for them; you are better off finding a club that is convenient, and offers a flat fee up front for a fixed period of time with no charges for fitness classes (yoga, Pilates, spinning, aerobics, etc.). ⟵

Let's return to our story before our pudgy protagonist gets grumpier and his rump gets even rumpier.

Harry has an epiphany (and takes three ibuprofens).

Now, where were we? Oh yeah, Muscles is a wee bit wary of that roly-poly in the ridiculous Bogart hat. And, Harry is checking out Muscles, thinking to himself, "Just look at that smug mug and the brazen way he shows off for his fabulously firm fan club. This guy's so gung-ho, he probably hands out steroids for Halloween. Just look at him flexing his forearms, his lats, and his traps. Well, I have set a nice little trap for you!"

Meanwhile, Muscles darts a glimpse at the overweight primate in the alligator shoes, thinking, "Look at that character out of a film noir B-movie. He's so dense, he probably thinks Gatorade is a music festival to save Florida's reptiles. Too bad it couldn't save the ones on his feet."

Now, Rip the trainer pops up in Harry's face. "Okay," he says, towing Harry to a row of stationary bikes. "Before I show you the ropes, I want you to loosen up a little." He slaps the bicycle seat. "Get up here and peddle awhile, about ten or fifteen minutes."

Harry throws a pudgy leg over the bike and (ooooch!) thwacks his sizeable testes on the pointy part of the seat.

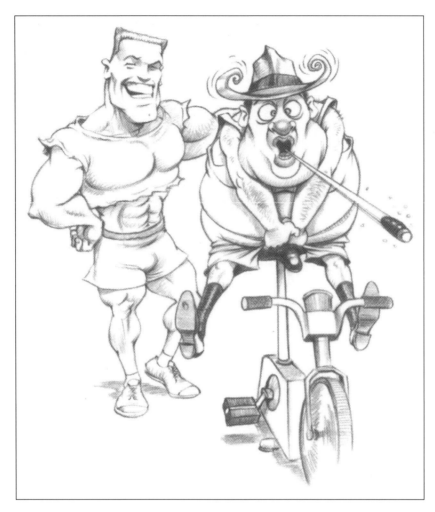

OUCH

On the Bike

While Harry is grimacing, a reminder that you should always adjust the seat first. And, unless you take pleasure in a foot cramp, never pedal with your toes.

"What are all these gizmos?" Harry asks, pointing to all the bells and whistles on the bike, the flashing red dots and beeping green arrows.

"This one right here?" Rip says, pointing to a digital counter. "It tells you how many calories you are burning. So burn, baby, burn!"

Harry croaks, "If I don't die of a heart attack, I will probably die of boredom."

"You can watch TV," Rip offers, pointing to a row of television sets. "Or, you can pass the time reading this fine literature," handing Harry a mucky, sweat-soaked tabloid.

Harry spins his wheels and laughs as he reads the *Irrational Inquirer*, while keeping a stealthy eye on Muscles. [4]

Attention English lit fans: here are a few of the smutty, libelous headlines that had Harry chuckling:

- Shocking Discovery! Schwarzennegger Can't Spell His Own Name

- Workouts Cause Cancer! Scientists Disclose that Sugar is Good for You in Large Doses

- Astonishing Revelation! Guys Tell Lies to Have Sex

- Boy has X-Ray Eyes! Banned from World Gym

- Girl, 13, Hears Wedding Bells! Parents Have Her Ears Removed

- Butcher Sells Own Tongue to Pay for Daughter's Operation! Hero Sandwich Heralded

- Woman Loses 283 Lbs. on Mouse Diet! "Secret is avoiding late night snacks," purrs successful dieter

- Girl with Halitosis Terrorizes Town! Lawyer Pleads Garlic Defense

- Aliens Without Green Cards! The Real Truth Why UFOs Never Landed

Harry peddles along, reading smut and spying on Marinara, while also eavesdropping on neighboring cyclists who are chattering and peddling away.

Personal Trainers

If a fitness instructor tells you to push through the pain, beware while you are burning, baby, beware! Of the approximately six million Americans who seek personal training in a year, a small yet alarming percentage end up seeking medical attention. Anyone can put out a shingle (not the shingles) with no experience required. Personal trainer wannabes can jump on the internet, fork out a few bucks for a textbook and an exam and—presto!—get a certificate in the mail before you can say Rip (OFF) Van Ripple. —

---

[4]Anything that encourages you to move is good, except maybe running from the law or a grizzly bear, which can run the length of a football field in six seconds. Nonetheless, you won't see many of them in the NFL. They can't catch a pigskin worth a darn, even with those razor-sharp claws. Eat it, yes. Catch it, no.

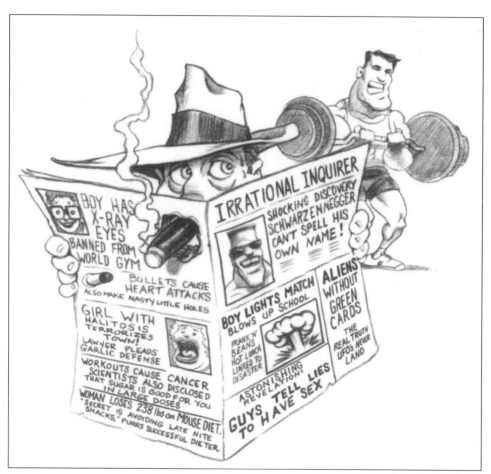

HARRY IS ALL EYES AND SMOKE

Says one, "If wine is too young, is that statutory grape?"

And, some Seinfeld wannabe says, "Why is it when you are in a movie theater, you can laugh as loud as you want, but if you whisper, people shush you?"

Someone else asks, "What about herpes II? What is that? A sequel?"

"This place is a regular laugh riot," grumbles Harry as he keeps an eye on Marinara, who is still there, beaming and bulging. Harry turns back to the Inquirer for another weird headline:

Deranged Youth Slays Man with Boiled Chicken! Police Suspect Fowl Play

One of the cyclists starts yapping about aging gracefully, to which some pedaling yoyo yaks back, "You call being injected,

Liposuction

Lazy gut-busters sometimes resort to liposuction, especially if they hate love handles. Rather than sucking in that stomach, they would rather have it sucked away. Local anesthesia is required and serious complications, although rare, can be life threatening. Look for a doctor who has performed as many liposuctions as Liz Taylor has had husbands. A good lipo-sucking costs thousands of dollars. Hmmm…crunches anyone? ——

implanted, augmented, and lipo-sucked to death 'aging gracefully'?" Replies Miss Aging Gracefully, "I know a doctor who will give you full pouty lips for five hundred bucks."[5]

Harry thinks, "You want full, pouty lips? I'll sock you in the kisser for fifty bucks."

While the chatty cyclists babble about toned biceps and blissful quadriceps, the chitchat is making Harry irritable, and the more irritable he gets, the faster he peddles.

All this prattling about sculpting and gulping, stress reduction and rear reduction is starting to bug the heck out of Harry, until finally he tears off two little pieces of newspaper, crumples them into teeny balls and shoves them into his ears. That's when he realizes how wet they are—not just his ears, but every part of his whopping anatomy is

dripping wet. And all this pouring sweat, damn, it feels good to him, although he is breathing hard. Not only has his breathing become difficult, his heart is beginning to sound like that Iron Butterfly drum solo in "Inna Godda Davida" (boom-boom-boppidy-boom-boom-bobbidy).

Fringe Benefits

Riding a bike is not only a good cardio-vascular workout, it also improves your quads and glutes, not to mention your endurance—even Harry's. ——

Check Yourself Out

To determine your maximum target heart rate: men subtract your age from 220; women subtract your age from 226. Figure your target rate zone by calculating 50% or 85% of maximum (almost as easy to figure out a waiter's gratuity).

For example, Harry is 40 years old: 220 - 40 = 180. 180 x 50% = 90, at the low end of the target zone or, 180 x 85% = 153, at the high end. If Harry takes his pulse for six seconds and counts thirteen beats and adds zero, he gets 130 for one minute, his target. Keep in mind, these are just estimates. ——

---

[5]After the actress, Barbara Hershey, had collagen injections in her lips for her role in the movie, *Beaches*, a fad was born: pouty lips. Talk about your Hershey Kisses!

Harry's heart rate tips you off to why you should consult a doctor before beginning a new workout regime. When you see your doctor, first, he checks you out, then he makes you write a check.

With his heart thumping—boom-boom-boppidy-boom-boom-bobbidy—Harry wisely slows down and gets off the bike, looking apprehensively over at the treadmill. Mind-numbing, treadmills are; blank minds walking nowhere. He sluggishly gets on it and, while lumbering along at two miles an hour, he goes back to trying to read that soggy, smutty tabloid.

Next thing he knows, he is lying on the floor, looking up at a broad-shouldered mug with a flat, boxer's nose. "Are you okay?" asks Muscles Marinara, his square face gazing down at Harry's round one.

"Yeah, pal, I'm fine and dandy," whispers Harry. In fact, Harry was dehydrated. He needed water. Maybe he also needed the U.S. Cavalry, but likely, he needed leg elevation, fresh air, and certainly, more water.

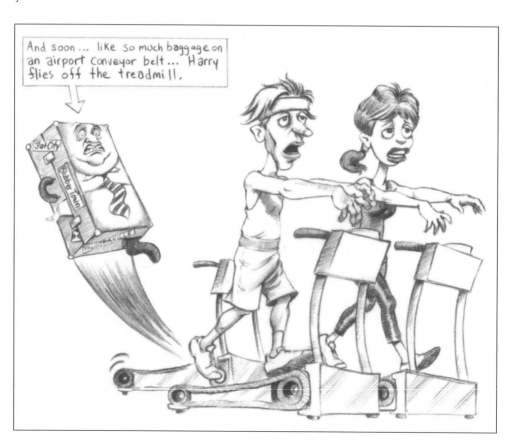

Strength

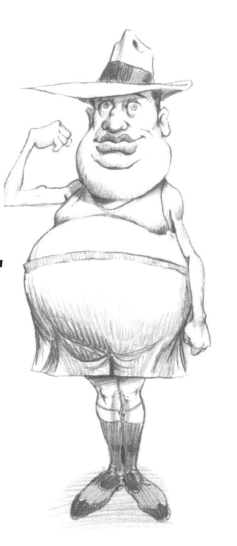

Bankruptcy

Oops, sorry.

Wrong Chapter Seven. Forget Chapter Seven.

Let's scoot along to Chapter 8.[1]

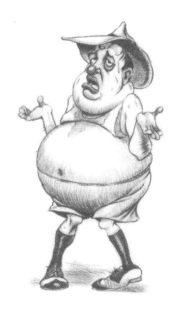

---

[1]Not to be confused with scat. Cats scat, people scoot. And, nothing burns calories quite like a good scoot.

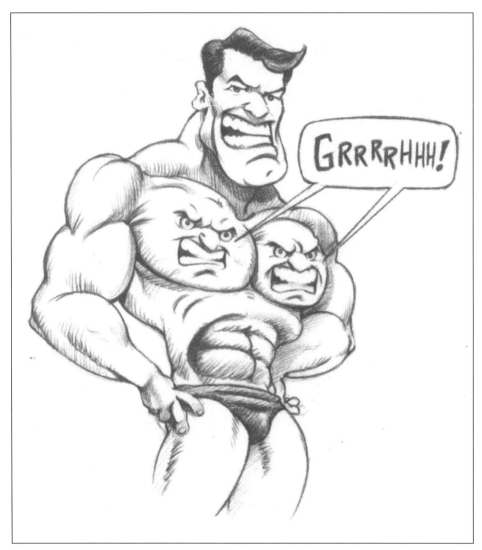

Don't Pec on Me

Everything You Want to Know About Pecs...

...But Are Too Intimidated to Ask

When we left Harry, he was lying on the gym floor looking up at Muscles Marinara. Little cartoon birdies chirped and twittered and flapped their cute widdle wings as they whirled around and around Harry's hazy head. My, what a lovely opportunity to talk pecs.

As mentioned briefly in Chapter Six, the pectoralis major and minor, commonly referred to as pectorals, comprise a muscle group that, when fully developed, can give a man the kind of cleavage that rivals Anna Nicole-Smith's. A deep, well-defined chest is one of the most important parts of the body for enhancing the appearance of a body-builder. Strong pectoral development increases the mass of the muscles, developing both "heads" of the pectoral muscles, deepening the groove between the two heads and creating a dip in the midline to give the impression of great bulk—a two-headed monster, so to speak.[1]

There is a new pecking order in gyms. It's called pecs. But, you don't need a gym to get them. You don't necessarily need weights or machines to get this groovy grooved effect. In fact, you don't need a damned thing, except a mirror (see below). The advantages are obvious. You can observe your form and technique, admire your ever-increasing muscle mass, and every now and then, apply a little lip gloss.

Mighty Mass

Got a mirror? Good. Sit in front of it and suck in your tummy, raising your arms even with your shoulders. Bend them at the elbows and flex your biceps like you are Mighty Mouse on cheesy steroids.

---

[1] Even though this muscle group is called the pectorals, they have other names, including the meatles. You may recall their debut album, *Beat the Meatles*, which featured their smash single, "I Wanna Hold Your Hamstring."

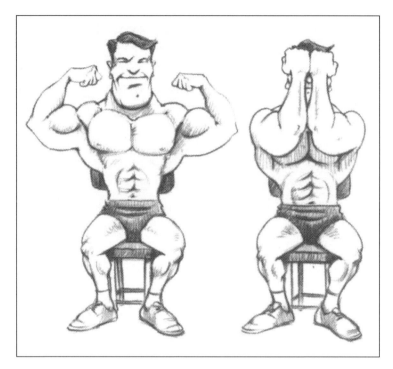

Pec Out - Pec In

Now, leading with your elbows...wait! Mice don't have elbows! Okay, so you can flex your biceps like the Incredible Hulk or King Kong.

That's it! Flex 'em like King Kong! And, imagine that you are holding in each enormous hairy hand a teensy-weensy little blonde who is kicking and screaming.

Getting back to leading with your elbows...bring your forearms together in front of your face (careful not to mangle your nose, Cyrano), contracting and squeezing your whole upper body as your elbows come together. Repeat this over and over until your chest screams, "Uncle!" and your arms scream, "Medic!" Do this Mighty Mass exercise whenever you can, wherever you can, day after day, until your pecs are perfect; or should I say, pecfert?

The Mighty Mass can be utterly boring, so try doing it to music. Keep it up and your pecs will swell, and you will have swell pecs the size of Chevy hubcaps.

HINT...

When working on your pecs at a gym, wear a Walkman or carry an MP3 player. If you are reading this in the year 2093, turn up your surgically implanted surround sound.

Another way to pare your pecs without weights, equipment, or a gym is by a process known as isometrics. Iso means, "I so sore," and metrics means, "My pecs so sore they grew a meter."

Isometrics is resistance exercise involving muscle contraction through pushing and pulling against an immovable object (such as Dom DeLuise, not to be confused with Dom Perignon, a moveable object filled with a bubbly substance that, when poured repeatedly into your date's cut crystal flute, makes him or her immovable).

Resistance exercise is also known as dynamic tension, a type of activity that has turned many a 97-pound weakling into a perfectly (or pecfertly) developed specimen just like the he-man, Charles Atlas.

For fifty years, Atlas sold millions of his exercise programs; you can still buy one at www.charlesatlas.com.

Synonymous with strength, Atlas was a household word. In his sixties, he pulled a 145,000-pound railroad car more than 120 feet with a rope. His name conjures up images of manly muscles in bright-white, ultra-tight briefs (his signature attire), and a deep, dark suntan that even George Hamilton would kill for (if melanoma doesn't kill him first).

His dynamic resistance method has weathered time, two World Wars and even the stock market crash of 1929. It may even survive the influx of health clubs and gyms, free weights, and Nautilus and Cybex training equipment.

Mr. Atlas

Now a part of American folklore is the story of Charles Atlas, who in the 1920s transformed himself from a 97-pound weakling into a "real man" through what he termed "dynamic tension," or isometrics. In 1922, Atlas was awarded the title, "World's Most Perfectly Developed Man." He came up with ads featuring a skinny nerd who swears revenge after getting sand kicked in his face by a beach-blanket bully. With the Charles Atlas muscle-building kit, the guy turns into a buffed hunk and attracts girls at the beach. ⎯

Here is a testimonial letter from one of Atlas' many satisfied specimens.

"The muscles of my chest stand out like a pair of 400-pound albinos posing with the Honorable Elijah Muhammad. My muscles are so big and hard that even Janet Reno is giving me the eye. I have achieved better results in a short time of doing isometrics in the privacy of my home than in ten years at the gym. I can't wait until some Left Coast latte liberal kicks a little sand in my face. I'll kick his bleeding heart from Hyannisport to the Hamptons!"

–D. Cheney, District of Columbia

The Chair Crunch
(also known as the Pygmy Push)

Here is a simple dynamic tension exercise to turn your toy chest into a strongbox. It requires only patience, perseverance, and

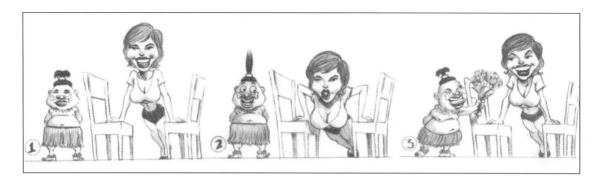

two chairs. If you reside in the Amazon rainforest, are not yet extinct, and cannot find a couple of chairs, a couple of friendly pygmies will do fine.

Before political correctness and strict immigration laws were imposed, some people used sedated pygmies for this exercise. Since you probably do not reside in the rainforest and you have a sense of human decency, kindly grab your chairs and place them about a foot and a half apart.

Rest your hand on top of each head; er... I mean chair. Your arms should be straight and your body extended in a sloping position, toes on the floor.

Keeping your body rigid, bend your elbows, dipping as low as you can between the chairs, getting your chest as near to the floor as possible. Now, do a push-up.[2] Repeat until slightly pooped.

Try to do this at least 100 times a day in sets of 10 or 20. If you are unable to do this, either you are a wimp, or you have a life.

Remember as you perform any tension-filled, face-twisting muscle maneuvers, take care not to make contorted faces.

My mother, a noted expert on twisted, contorted facial expressions, says your face will become wrinkled at an early age if you frown. She has experimented with Botox and—oops—her face is now frozen into an expression of disaffection and perpetual boredom, which is an improvement over the expression of general displeasure that formerly gripped her features.

Be warned! One little slip with Botox can lead to you looking like you have suffered from a minor stroke.

Pec Potentiality

Big pecs are big business. For example, don't be surprised if film festivals finally pay tribute to Gregory Pec. And, expect some genius to invent a tool to dislodge food trapped in cleavages, calling it "toothpecs," while some brainy brewery comes up with Six-Pecs.

---

[2]You don't have to be Al Einstein (or Mel Einstein) to realize this is just doing push-ups between two chairs. It made Chuck E. Atlas a rich man, and does it ever perk up the pecs!

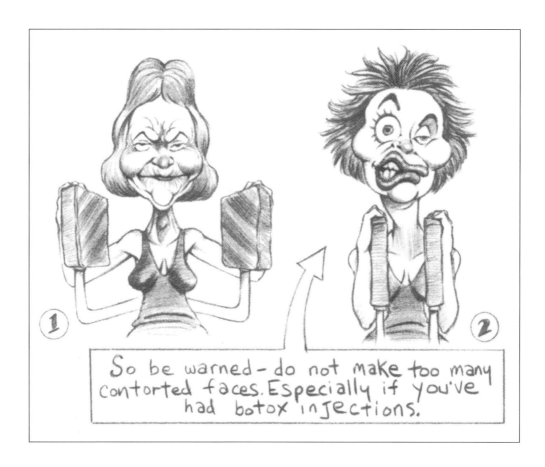

Pecs and Peccadillos

There are many ways to build up your pecs. Most of them you will not find within these pages. There is bench-pressing, which stretches the entire pectoral mass, particularly the outer and lower sections of the muscle. And you can also use the incline press, the decline press, and the calvinklein press.

If you are too lazy to go through all this hard work to have a hard he-man or she-woman chest, go to a surgeon and have your pecs implanted. Is that cheating? If you compete for Mr. Universe, yes. For Ms. Universe? Nah.

A Sorely Needed Sit-Up

Part Four

The broad-shouldered, square-jawed Muscles Marinara gazes down at the rotund face of Harry Potbelly, while the adorable, hard body seductress with the washboard abdomen, Theresa Triathlon, caresses one of the many Marinara bulges.

"Aha!" thinks Harry. "Caught you two red handed!" Harry staggers to his feet and is about to pull out his subminiature surveillance camera, the one he keeps hidden under his fedora, when that wonder of a woman, Mrs. Muscles—Monica Marinara—sashays into the gym.

"Oh boy, oh boy, oh boy," he thinks. "This is gonna be one helluva showdown."

"Hi Toots," Harry says to Monica, as he points a plump and clammy finger at the finely-chiseled Jezebel whose hands are all over Muscles' muscles. "Miss Triathlon here is the femme fatale that is trying to steal your husband."

Muscles says to Harry, "You must have bumped your head hard when you fell off the treadmill because I have no idea what you are blathering about."

"Heh-heh," Harry heh-hehs, giving Mrs. Muscles a conspiratorial wink. "I'm sure your wife Monica here and her trusty team of attorneys will gladly explain it to you in divorce court."

Flexing every muscle in his pecs, delts, biceps, and the long striated cords of his back—you name it, it's flexed, Muscles says, "That's not my wife. I'm not even married."

Harry reels back as if a missile has screamed down from unfriendly skies, crashed through the ceiling of Rick's Gym and put a cleft in his cranium.

"A stud like me?" sniggers Muscles. "Married? That's a good one, and it makes as much sense as packing snowshoes for a Mexican holiday."

"Okay, pal," Harry says while aiming a stubby finger at Monica. "Who is this woman?"

Muscles splutters, "I have no idea, pal." Giving the curvaceous Monica a smile so

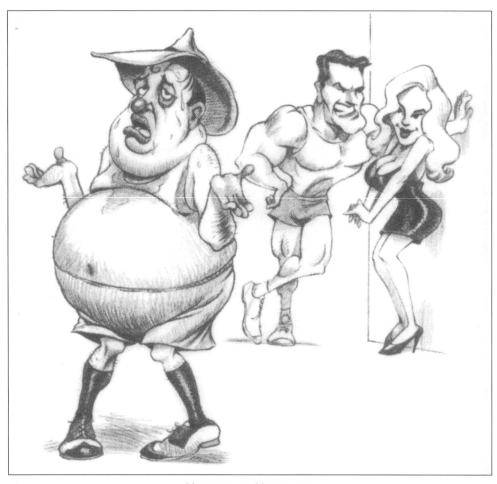

MATCHMAKER, MATCHMAKER

radiant it could melt Antarctica, he adds, "I'm sure I'll have a ball finding out."

As Muscles and Monica become palsy-walsy, Harry is left standing there befuddled, sweat dripping off his pudgy, slack jaw, still feeling a little woozy from his spill off the treadmill. He looks over to see Dr. Linker step off a Stairstepper and walk over.

"Hi Harry," the Doc says. "This is all my fault. You see, knowing you are a great gumshoe, not to mention a very big one, I figured I'd get you to tail Muscles, knowing it would lead you into this gym. I hired the shapely thespian here to pose as Mrs. Marinara."

"She's an actress?" Harry gasps.

"Yep, I hired her to hire you to get you to follow him so he would lead you here."

"But…"

"Butt!" the Doc says. "That's what it's all about, your big butt, and your beer belly. Remember, Harry, how you rescued me years ago? Well, now it's my turn to rescue you. You are over forty, right? With all that smoking, drinking, saturated fat, and lack of exercise, you will be lucky to make it to fifty. I am trying to pay you back, Harry."

Just then, the personal trainer, Rip Van Ripple, pokes his puss over the Doc's shoulder and blurts, "Don't worry, Doc, I'll whip him into shape."

"No, you won't, Rip," says the Doc, "Harry needs a lot of TLC. Theresa, he's all yours."

And the woman Harry thought was a Jezebel, the one who gave him a belly full of butterflies now gives Harry a pearly-white, sexy smile. "Don't you worry," she says. "I'll give Harry nothing but some very tender, loving, personal training."

"Hmmm," thinks Harry. "This is one trainer with whom I plan to get very personal."

Okay, Harry," Theresa says. "Reel in your tongue and put your eyes back in their sockets. Follow me to the hard-rubber floor mat. It's crunch time!"

"Crunches?" says Harry. "I do those all the time." Taking out a partially melted Nestle Crunch bar, he adds with a grin, "I've been doing Crunches for years. Once I did forty-three Crunches in one sitting. I had to stop because I got a terrible toothache."

Theresa Teaches Harry to Crunch

"Pay attention to your form and technique," Theresa says. "And I'll show you how to really crunch. First, lie on your back with your knees bent. Put your hands anywhere you want, except on me. Some people cross them over the chest; some relax them beside the head. I like putting them behind my head.

"Take care not to interlace your fingers as that can pull on your neck and use arm strength rather than your abs. The more you pull on your head, the less effective the crunch.

"Now, Harry, contract your abs. No, not that kind of contract. No signing on the dotted line, just squeezing those muscles nice and tight. Good, Harry! Don't forget to breathe, and focus, Harry, focus, not on the ceiling, on the contraction! Imagine you are pulling your rib cage towards your hipbone. Let that contraction pull your shoulders, chest, and shoulder blades slowly off the floor.

"And, take that ridiculous hat off, Harry! Ooooh, what a cute little camera you have there," Theresa says. "Rip, come over here and show Harry how to do a crunch."

She goes on, "Okay, Harry, now your upper body is about halfway to an upright position, about six to twelve inches off the floor. Hold that contraction. Gooooood!

"Now, while you inhale, lower yourself slowly to the floor. Even if you are a former

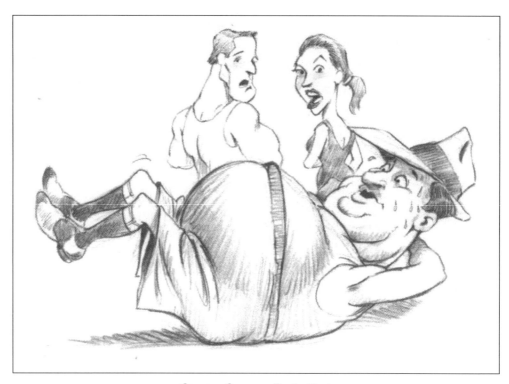

Crunch, Crunch—Do It, Do It

smoker you have permission to inhale. And, I hope you are a former smoker, Harry. I hate the thought of kissing someone who tastes like an ashtray. Remember, you are doing the work, not gravity. Lower yourself slowly.

"When your head touches the floor, don't relax–tighten your contraction and do it again and again and again, until you are really pooped.

"Now, that wasn't so bad, was it?" she asks. Harry is panting like a puppy.

Ignoring his dribble, Theresa says, "Good, Harry. Ready for another set?"

Harry is not ready.

"Don't worry," she giggles. "We will take this one day at a time. No, make that one minute at a time, one measly sit-up, followed by another and another. Those minutes add up, so whether your goal is three minutes or three sit-ups, you will attain your goal. Just do it, do it, do it."

With Theresa by his side, all Harry has on his mind is doing it.

After Harry showers off and catches his breath, Dr. Linker gives him a congratulatory high five. "Harry," he says "You helped me once. Now, you're on your way to better health."

Flopping a flabby arm around the Doc's shoulder, like Bogey at the end of *Casablanca*, Harry says, "Doc, I think this is the beginning of a healthy friendship. And,

Abs, Abs and More Abs

Note that sit-ups, crunches, and other abdominal exercises will strengthen your muscles, although you may not see a washboard stomach until you get rid of the fat on top of it. Muscle replaces abdomen fat, and it may not decrease your abdomen size. You will lose weight only by using more calories than you take in. Exercise and eat a healthy diet, replacing junk food with fruits and veggies (see Section III, Diet).

it may be the beginning of a heck of a gym relationship."

They laughed and headed out the door into the evening fog, while the Doc continued his unsolicited lecture series about exercise.

"Listen up, Harry. Exercise reduces the risk of colon cancer; helps you sleep more soundly; lowers cholesterol and burns calories. Just remember to stay away from saturated fat—animal fats in meat and dairy products (yes, in chopped liver). These fats play a role in raising cholesterol levels and increasing the risk of cardiovascular disease.

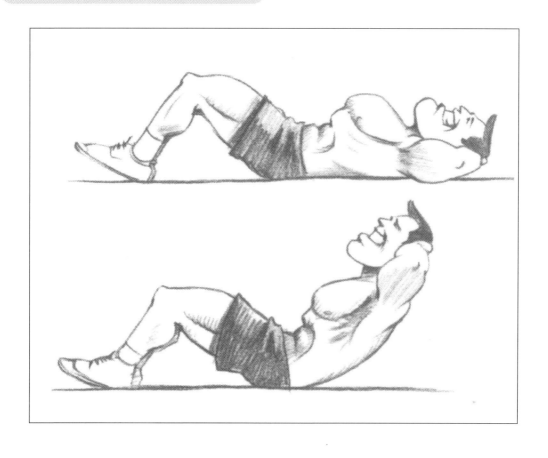

"And another big advantage for you," offers the Doc, "is if you are in good physical shape, when you're on the prowl, you'll have a better chance with the gym society. Gyms are havens for honeys." (If you are a honey, think of this: 'Hunks Ahoy!')

Giving the Doc a wave, Harry walks away, slowly disappearing into the night. Just about everybody at Rick's Gym and the Doc, too, have good feelings that Harry Potbelly is well on his way to becoming Harry Six-Pack, Harry Yoked, maybe even Harry Washboard.

Workouts of the Rich and Flabby

How to Go From Rich and Aspiring to Bitchy and Perspiring

Hey there, you with this book in your face. Are you reading this while pedaling on a stationary bike? Or while lying on the sofa? If you are among the rich and flabby, chances are you are in the market for a short workout, a little toning to go with your tanning.

If everyone gets fifteen minutes of fame, you certainly have fifteen minutes to zap some of your fabulous flab. You may be too busy making money hand over flaccid fist to squeeze in a long workout, but a quickie you can always find time for.

Number one, get some designer apparel to go with your YSL sweatshirt and your Manolo sneakers. I recommend Donatella Versace, Gucci, or Valentino because even your sweat should smell expensive. Aaah, that sweet smell of success—the champagne wishes, the caviar dreams, the Prada yada yada.

To stay toned so you can continue to fit into your designer duds, I recommend stretching out your muscle groups. This will prevent injury and keep your innards taut, and your ligaments lubricated. Before you stretch, warm up for five minutes by cycling gently or running in place. Keep in mind that stretching too much too soon—unless you are naturally limber—can cause injury.

A typical warm-up exercise for the rich and flabby once went like this:

- Put on cashmere sweater.

- Turn thermostat way up.

  The typical cool-down was:

- Take off cashmere sweater.

- Turn air conditioner way up.

Stretch

Not just for Slinkys and saltwater taffy, stretching is a must before and after a workout to reduce the risk of injury, soreness, and cramps. ◂

That was then, this is now. You can warm up by walking, cycling or spinning, before starting Thai kickboxing, Tae-Bo, Ju-Jitsu, Karate, Aikido, Tai Chi Kuan, and the other thirty-one flavors like yoga, Pilates and gyrotonics.

Clawing to the Top

If you suffer from a Karma Deficit Disorder, here is an exercise that is great for your quads and hamstrings.

- Go halfway up a ladder (a social ladder is fine).

- Kiss the ass above you while kicking the face below.

- Repeat 8 to 12 times, slowly.

- Watch your form: always kiss up and kick down; up, down, up, down. Be sure to wear enough Chapstick.

The Gates Workout

Here is another quickie workout for the rich and flabby that takes no more than fifteen minutes, give or take a nanosecond (or a nanny).

Anyone with fifty billion bucks can buy a little time, and an old gate. If Bill Gates had bought time to do this exercise, his company might now be called Microfirm instead of...soft.

- Go to Christie's auction house and make the highest bid for the classic wrought-iron gate used in the opening scenes of the movie, *Citizen Kane*.

- Lift the gate 8 to 12 times.

- Repeat until your heart rate resembles the Nasdaq composite (on the downside).

The Case Workout

The former Chairman of AOL Time Warner, Steve Case, may not be flabby, yet hanging out with all those rock bands is beginning to expand his waistband. If you want a billionaire's belly, try the Case Workout:

- Get a case of imported beer.

- Lift a bottle to your lips.

- Chug until empty.

- Repeat until case is empty, or until acquired (and don't forget to squeeze traps, lats, and net profits).

- Return the empties.

The Donald Workout

Donald Trump took over his daddy's business and established himself as one of the world's flabbiest developers. He developed everything from hotels to casinos, everything, that is, except muscles.

To get a set of The Donald's underdeveloped muscles for yourself, do this:

- Pick up dumb blondes.

- Lift blondes 8 to 12 times each and repeat until bankrupt and/or divorced, whichever comes first.

The Famous Fifteen

Here is a fifteen-minute workout that requires a stationary bike and a pair of light weights (or a couple of bulging wallets) weighing 3-5 pounds each.

- First, warm up for one minute by peddling on the bike at a moderate speed while holding the weights at your sides. Now, pedal for another minute while doing as many shoulder presses as you can.

- Next, for another minute, hold the weights down at your sides and speed up your pedaling, then slow down for a minute while doing as many seated rows as you can.

- For one more minute, speed up your pedaling while holding the weights down at your sides. Now, slow your pedaling for one minute while doing as many lateral raises as you can.

- For one minute, speed up pedaling while holding the weights down at your sides; then, for another minute, slow-pedal and do as many tricep extensions as you can.

- Again, hold the weights down at your sides while speeding up your pedaling for one minute. Now, for one minute, slow-pedal while doing as many bicep curls as you can.

How To..

Shoulder press: bend your arms so that the weights are on either side of your head at ear level. Extend your arms to press the weights overhead.

Seated rows: hold the weights with your arms extended in front of your body just below breast level. Pull your arms back while squeezing shoulder blades together.

Lateral raise: starting with the weights down at your sides, raise arms straight out to the sides to shoulder level.

Tricep extension: while holding the weights, raise your arms overhead, bend your elbows so your hands are behind your head. Slowly straighten your arms overhead, keeping upper arms close to the sides of your head.

Bicep curls: hold your arms straight down by your sides, palms facing forward. Keeping your elbows close to your body, bend your arms to bring the weights toward your chest. —

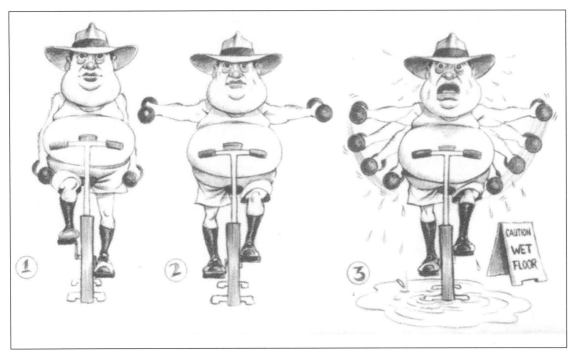

LATERAL RAISE

● Speed up your pedaling again while holding the weights down at your sides. Whew! Now, take a moment to towel off—and wring it out!

● Ready for some push-ups? Do as many as you can in one minute. Do them either from your toes or, if you have a troublesome back, from your knees. Go!

● Now, roll over and do three minutes of crunches (review Chapter 9 for correct crunches).

Your fifteen minutes are up, rich and flabby fans. You are muscle enriched!

Good Lord, Get a Grip!

Dumbbells for Dummies

If your idea of lifting is raising a martini, you have another thing coming (or another drink coming). Lifting weights is more than just building biceps; it also improves cardiovascular fitness.

Weight lifting and muscle building is sometimes called strength training, because—duh—it makes you stronger.[1]

The stronger you are, the more active you can become; and the more active you are, the stronger you are—a marvelous cycle. So, let's go cycling! Or dancing, or canoeing, or hopscotching. Whatever you do, lifting weights will give you the energy to do it. And, all it takes is a couple of dumbbells, which are as cheap as bananas, and far less squishy.

You may opt to join a fitness club and use their equipment. Using their dumbbells is what I recommend because there is less chance of stubbing your toe on one when you race to the bathroom in the middle of the night.

Using Weights for Strength Training

Before the advent of strength training, a weight was something used to hold paper down on a desk. Now, just try to find a good paperweight. I use a Tom Waits CD as a paperweight—you could call it a Tomweight.

Today, weights are things that slip onto a bar and make you grunt, grimace, and groan; things that make some people look like Superman, and some like the Michelin Man.

You lift weights. You curl them, press them, and curse them. And, you gotta love them. Governor Ah-nold does, and he will be the first to tell you that the veights can't vait. Take it slow-ly, and focus on form and

---

[1]Strength training is not to be confused with trength straining. Nothing is more painful than a strained trength. Because I don't know what a trength is, I wouldn't want to strain it.

technique for less risk of injuries and greater chance of success.

Get a grip, and lift! Here is something to mull over: if weight lifting is now called strength training, shouldn't dumbbells be called smartbells? And what about the small, light, hand weights; shouldn't they be called Tinkerbells?

Speaking of lifting, if you would like to read an uplifting tale, lift the corner of this page...and turn.

Weighty Wisdom...

Weights are available in all sizes and styles including chrome, Neoprene, and gabardine (okay, maybe not gabardine, but a thick, rugged corduroy would be nice). Hex weights are one of the simplest, cheapest types of dumbbells you can buy. Cast from iron and coated with baked enamel, they are hexagonal in shape to avoid rolling, so you will not have to chase them down six flights of stairs while waking up your crotchety landlady.

Drop Sets

Drop sets: no, this doesn't mean dropping a set of weights on your foot. Dropping a set of weights means reducing the weight by about 30%. Choose a weight you can hoist 4 to 6 times, then lift until the brink of failure.

Now, without taking a breather, remove 30% of the weight and repeat. Follow immediately with one more drop set, again dropping weight so it's about 30% lighter. Perform these reps slowly: three counts up, three counts down. When you complete your drop sets, rest for about two minutes, then go on to another exercise. Crunches and push-ups, or twist-twist-twisting to open bottles of ibuprofen.

The Three Ripped Pigs

And other Curly Short Tales about Curling that will have you Huffin' and Puffin'

The following conversation between a Mr. Wolf and a Miss Piggy took place at the Gorilla Sports Gym, which, you may recall, is a great place for animals to congregate.

Says Miss Piggy, who is doing a bicep curl, "You sort of remind me of Prince."

Replies Mr. Wolf, with a huff and a puff as he does a military press, "You mean Prince, the Artist Formerly Known As?"

"No, not that Prince," Piggy sniggers as she does a set of preacher curls.

Doing a bent-arm barbell pullover, and with that big toothy grin of his, Mr. Wolf asks, "Prince Andrew of Windsor?"

"No, not that Prince," replies Miss Piggy, while thinking to herself, "Oh my, what big lats you have!"

Mr. Wolf, more curious than ever, asks, "Prince Albert of Monaco?"

"Nope," says Miss Piggy, while thinking, "Oh my, what big delts you have!"

With a snicker, she lowers the weight and the boom. "Just some mangy mutt named Prince I used to own," she says. "He got so...I had to put him to sleep."

The wolf growls. He isn't such a bad wolf, otherwise he would have pigged out on Miss Piggy by now.

Jim Gorilla, the personal trainer, cautiously approaches the predator, praying not be preyed upon. "I hope I'm not being too nosy, Mr. Wolf," he says. "But do you still huff and puff when you blow houses down?"

"That is all in the past," the wolf snorts, his long snoot dripping sweat, as he gently places the dumbbells back in the rack. "I am a born-again canis lupus, which means I huff and puff only when lifting weights, and only for effect."

For muscles to get stronger, they must be continually challenged. Once your body makes the necessary adjustments, after about 8 to 12 weeks of exercise, dramatic muscle change levels off.

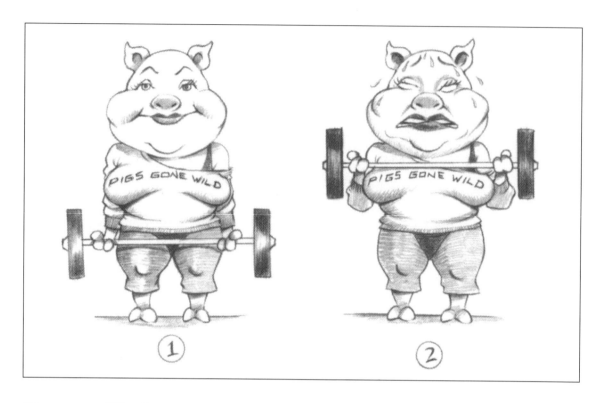

Dummy Up I

Bicep curl: with feet (or hooves) planted hip-width apart, grasp barbell, holding arms straight down by your sides. Keeping upper arms close to body, bend elbows to curl forearms to chest and upper arms. Slowly lower to starting position. Try to do 2 sets of 12 reps without oinking or smelling like bacon grease. (See above.)

Military press: with feet (or rear paws) hip-width apart, grasp barbell (a wolf calls it barkbell), positioning hands at shoulder height. Slowly straighten overhead; lower to starting position. Try to do 2 sets of 12 reps without getting that bushy tail stepped on (or devouring someone's grandma). (See page 74.)

For continued muscle growth, and to keep burning fat, alternate lighter weight workouts with heavier ones, every couple of weeks. Also, wearing a skin-tight Jim Skinz muscle shirt will give you the appearance of being more cut (unless you happen to have a very furry chest like Mr. Wolf).

"Careful you don't huff and puff too much, Mr. Wolf," Jim says. "It may be a sign that you are wolfing down the wrong diet."

"I no longer dig swine," says the wolf. "I now have a more nutritional diet."

HINT...

You are smart, Mr. Wolf, because leafy vegetables, particularly spinach and kale, are good sources of dietary fiber; protein; vitamins A, C, and B-complex; and minerals, especially calcium, iron, magnesium, and phosphorus. They are also low in carbohydrates and fats.

You don't think wolves eat plants? If plants can eat creatures (i.e., venus flytrap), then creatures can eat plants. For the record, wolves are carnivores, yet they eat other stuff, including earthworms, grasshoppers, berries, and an occasional spinach salad with a sliced, hard-boiled egg white.

Dummy Up II

Preacher curls: sit on a preacher bench (if you don't have one, a rabbi bench will do). Grasp a dumbbell with an underhand grip, place the back of one arm down on the pad and raise the dumbbell until your forearm is perpendicular to the floor with the back of the upper arm remaining on the pad. Lower the dumbbell until your arm is fully extended; repeat.

Focus on squeezing your biceps for a peak contraction during each movement. Keep your abs tight to stabilize your body, and to prevent an untimely hernia.

Barbell Pullover: go ahead, Mr. Wolf, lie on a flat bench on your back, your pointy ears pointing toward the floor. With barbell at chest, resting in line with the hips, use a foot-wide hand grip, keeping elbows in.

Inhale (or inhuff) and lower weight over chest, then face, until barbell almost touches the floor behind your head. Exhale (or expuff) and pull weights back to chest. Do a set of eight to twelve, or until you are able to blow down a house of sticks (if you can blow down bricks, report to the Oval Office).

You need do only one set (8 to 12 reps) per exercise for toning, as long as you fatigue your muscle with that set. If not fatigued, do two more. —

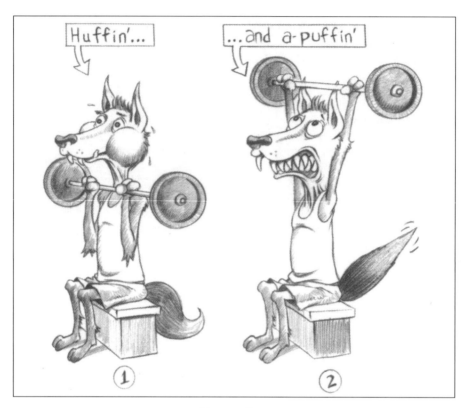

MILITARY PRESS

"Don't tell me you are now a big, bad vegan?" asks the trainer.

"I wouldn't go that far," says the wolf. "Now and then I like a bit of bacon over my kale."

Noticing Miss Piggy turn white, Mr. Wolf quickly amends, "Not to worry, Piss Miggy—I mean, Miss Piggy—I go for that faux bacon."

"Oh, facon!" Miss Piggy says. "Good." Returning to her normal pinkish glow, she adds, "Because I hate bit parts, especially bacon bit parts."

Gorilla, the trainer, says, "Now, instead of the Big Bad Wolf you are the Big Buffed Wolf?"

The wolf replies, "The more I curl and press, the buffer I get, and I am huffin' and puffin' a lot less, too."

"A heart isn't built with hay, sticks, or bricks," says Miss Piggy. "It is built with muscle and tissue, and a lot of willpower and discipline."

"Willpower is something I have," says Wolf. "If I didn't, Miss Piggy here would be pork chops by now."

With that, the little piggy went wee-wee-wee all the way home. And, the wolf howled.

Hansel and Pretzel

Unless you forgot to take your ginkgo biloba, you will recall that the wicked witch needed to fatten up Hansel and Pretzel. So what did she do? She stuffed the kids with saturated fats and sugar, then caged them so they couldn't exercise.

Smart little tykes, Hansel and Pretzel worked out while in the cage, doing sit-ups, push-ups,[1] running in place, and generally sweating like crazy. They even took turns lifting each other[2] to burn calories.

When the witch told them to stick out their fingers to see if they were nice and fat, she was dumbstruck to see they hadn't gained a single pound! Now, that is how you give a wicked witch the finger.

An Even Happier Ending

The witch was so hungry she flew to a fast-food restaurant where she stuffed her ugly face with greasy, fatty, deep-fried finger food. As her arteries were already clogged to capacity, she died of a coronary right on the spot—a grease spot. (Now you know why they call these fairy tales Grimm.)

As for the brother and sister trapped in a cage, because they had whipped themselves into such miraculous shape, busting out was a piece of cake with frosting—they escaped with all their fingers and toes intact.

Legend has it that Hansel's sister, who broke quite a sweat, is now a saltier Pretzel.

---

[1]You may have seen Jack LaLanne on TV doing push-ups with heavy objects on his back, such as a refrigerator. I do not advise placing a refrigerator on your back while doing your push-ups, for three reasons: it can hurt a lot; it can hurt a lot more; it can hurt so much you won't believe it. If Jack jumped off a bridge with a refrigerator on his back, would you do it? (Okay, maybe a small thermo-cooler or a refrigerator recently defrosted.)

[2]The great thing about lifting free weights is that each exercise can be altered by holding the weights in a different way: with palms facing forward, palms facing the thighs, palms facing the rear, or by facing the music, which is also facing the oven, if you happen to be in the same pickle as Hansel and Pretzel.

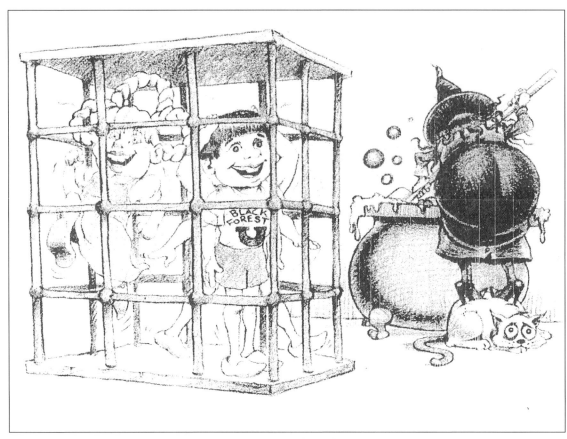

HANSEL AND PRETZEL'S FITNESS CENTER

Those Magnificent Machines

For the Upper Body, Lower Body, And Ain't Nobody

Yoked, chiseled, rock-hard, ripped. Chiclets, speedbumps, six-packs, washboards—these are just a few of the words that describe well-developed muscle mass. And, as you will learn in this chapter, it takes a mass of machinery to get muscle mass. Magnificent machines that hammer, clang, and bang out a rock-solid symphony of grunts and groans; a slogging, sweating tuneful of finely cut, highly toned musculature.

For some of you, those noisy, smelly, jam-packed gyms are a total turnoff. If so, you can dial one of those toll-free numbers (like 800-U-SUCKER or 800-RIPOFF) and order a tricky-to-assemble home gym that promises rock hard abs, sculpted legs, a well-toned physique, and a depleted bank account.

These TV-hyped muscle machines with names like Uglyflex or Fluxadux may come loaded with over 300 pounds of resistance, a lat tower, a low pulley/squat station, a leg extension/leg curl station, and a built-in adjustable pulley system. You may also get an absurdly overproduced instructional video that makes Cecil B. DeMille look like Cecil B. DeMilligram, and even a clothing rack for your workout duds (the latter being the most important feature since most of these Rube Goldbergian contraptions take up more closet space than Shaquille O'Neal).

Your other choice is to call Richard Simmons and invite him over: two for two, and two for toil? He will give you a far better workout than any of those pricey, non-weight-stack machines. And, Richard is easier on the eyes and so much easier to fold up and put away.

Before purchasing any exercise gear or hiring Richard, I suggest signing up for a short-term membership at a health club. It will have every machine you could ever need, plus trainers to show you how to clang and bang more efficiently.

Are there body-building machines for the brain? If there were, demand would outpace

HINT...

If the clanging and banging of all that machinery is giving you a big headache, find a health club that offers Pilates, a specialized set of exercises in which you work against your own body weight to develop strength and balance. Just say, "Puh-LAH-teez, puh-LEEZ!"

Use It or Lose It

If you do not use muscle, you lose muscle tone. But don't panic. Strength training just three times a week for thirty minutes increases the number of calories burned, enabling you to lose fat without losing muscle (as long as you don't spend the other four days pigging out, Miss Piggy). —

supply both near and far and in all sizes, shapes, and colors. There would also be a couple dozen in the nation's capital faster than you could say "weapons of mass destruction."

The Deltoid Machine

To build your shoulders and upper arms, it takes a minimal amount of brainpower. Sit comfortably, keeping your back firmly against the back support. Rest your feet either on the floor or on the footrest. Start with your arms bent, holding onto the weighted handles.

Keeping the same arm position, raise your arms up to shoulder level in a smooth motion, then lower slowly. Repeat.

Keep your arms in contact with the pads at all times. That way, you increase your domestic arms while, at the same time, reducing arms abroad.

Are there machines that spank? You wish, you naughty tramp. Getting flogged and thrashed is not everyone's cup of tedium. To avoid a potential spanking on the machines, move a pin and–voila!–you are lifting less weight. You can easily adjust strengthening machines to increase or decrease resistance...viva la resistance! This will produce a far less sadistic workout than, let's say, getting pinned under a heavy barbell.

Strength training may reduce the risk of heart disease, diabetes, and possibly colon cancer, and it may reduce the pain of arthritis and combat osteoporosis. This type of exercise also builds the major muscle groups—chest, shoulders, back, abdomen, arms, and legs—so you can hang out at nude beaches[1] (where there is a lot of flesh hanging out).

Stay away from steroids. Anabolic steroids can cause heart attacks, strokes, and liver problems. They can also cause undesirable body changes like breast development and genital shrinking in men. No way, Jose Canseco! Unless your

---

[1]Don't forget the sunscreen, or you will be more than just red in the face.

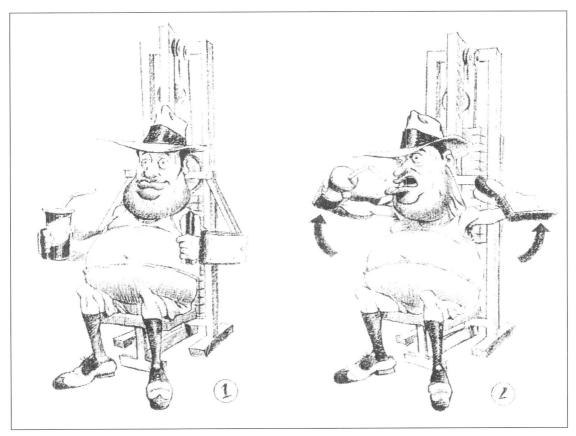

DELTOID WORKOUT

HINT...

Never Say in a Health Club:

- *"Pump fast, die young, leave a rock-hard corpse."*

- *"The path of a righteous man is beset on all sides by the iniquities of the selfish and the tyranny of evil men. And, I will strike down upon thee with great vengeance and furious anger those who do not wipe off their sweat!"*

- *"Thar she blows!"*

- *"I want my mommy!"*

- *"The mirrors are dirty!"*

- *"Steroids for sale!"*

- *"Gentleman, this is a bust... whatta bust!"*

name is Seabiscuit, why would you want to increase your muscle size at the risk of reducing the size of your genitals?

At The Gym

Don't let it all hang out. Wear shorts that are big enough; otherwise guys, they will find out you are not.

While on the road to fitness, avoid road rage. Do not throw a fit when someone forgets to pick up his or her sweat-soaked towel. Be courteous and polite; simply tell them where to stuff it (in the hamper, of course).

Don't just jump on a machine and start power pumping. Always check the adjustments, reinsert the pin, shift the seat up or down, and check the weight rack before you lift; otherwise, you may be racked, with pain.

Machines allow you to increase the resistance of an exercise, pushing you to the limit without the help of a spotter, which you may need with free weights. If you are prone to nosebleeds, you may need the help of a spot remover.

If you don't remember the name of a machine or how to use it, just ask a trainer.

Diet

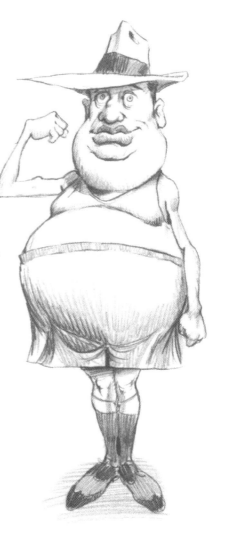

What to Eat, What NOT to Eat

And Stuff You Can Stuff

In a dog-eat-dog world, there are healthier things to eat than dog. Although some Native Americans once found dog a tasty treat, most of us now shy away from consuming anything that comes when called; or plays fetch, or rolls over and plays dead.

If you want to stay healthy and trim, here is the skinny— and it's not a greyhound.

Eat a low-fat diet. An alternate skinny is to eat a low-carbohydrate, high-fat diet, a la Dr. Atkins. Eat a diet that doesn't sit up and beg, or bark at you. After all, I am talking about roughage, not rrrufff-ruff.

Go for the Fiber Crunch

Roughage is fiber, and a low-fat diet high in fiber is the ideal.[1]

Fiber and weight management go hand-in-hand (or arm-in-arm, depending on whether they are dating or just good friends). High fiber foods take longer to chew and longer to digest, which means you will likely eat smaller portions and feel less hungry.

Insoluble Fiber

Indigestible by the human body, dietary fiber corrects disorders of the large intestine, like eensy-weensy Roto-Rooter men keeping things functioning normally. ◄

Fiber Snacks

Speaking of crunches, the next time you feel the urge to snack, grab high-fiber foods that crunch, such as carrots, apple slices, or jicama (which is Mexican minus the sombrero). ◄

---

[1]By fiber, I am not talking angora, I am talking flaxseed. Grind the seed—it is wonderful sprinkled on fruit or breakfast cereal. It's the seed that can help you become top-seeded!

More Fiber Snacks

Another way to cop a great fiber-rich snack is to enjoy a big bowl of minestrone, lentil, or split pea soup. You will fill up like a balloon from the soup, and the carbohydrates will release a brain chemical called serotonin that helps to create a natural high, like Gary Cooper in the movie, *High Noon*. (No, I have never heard of anyone smoking minestrone. Banana peels, yes…minestrone, no.) —

Food is one of life's greatest pleasures, right up there with having your back scratched or a good foot massage, or wiggling a Q-tip cotton swab into your ear and scooping out trapped wax. Entering the ear canal is not wise, since you can inadvertently puncture an eardrum or capsize a teeny gondolier. Haven't lost your appetite? Good, let's continue.

Even though they taste good, some foods are not good for us, often because they lack fiber. In the case of canned foods, the can may lie around too long, which may leach aluminum out of the tin and into the food.

What are Saturated Fats?

Other bad, bad foods are those drenched dangerously with tasty, saturated fat. Yucky, gooky, gum-glop that stimulates the production of LDL cholesterol (low density lipoprotein) is the bad guy that causes fatty plaques to build on the arterial wall, thereby increasing your risk of heart disease. If you were a cartoon, your eyes would go from 00s to XXs.

To put off meeting your maker for as long as possible, get the heck off LDL; it's a bad trip. Instead, get on HDL, which is high density lipoprotein, another way of saying monounsaturated fat (not to be confused with Minnesota Fats) and also polyunsaturated fats (not to be confused with Fats' wife, Polly).

HDLs are the good guys. Not only do they wear cute, microscopic white hats, they also reduce the risk of heart disease by carrying fat away from the arterial wall. You will find monounsaturated fats in many nuts, like almonds, cashews, and robinwilliams, and in olive and canola oils (not popeye oil), as well as avocados (not avamarias).

Let it be known that olive oil is a rich source of oleic acid, and you are hard-pressed (cold-pressed, in the case of the best quality olive oil) to find folks with heart disease in Mediterranean countries, where olive oil is king!

The Mediterranean diet is one of the healthiest in the world, according to statistics. Death rates from heart disease in such countries as Italy, Spain, and Greece are much lower than in the United States, where butter is the most common condiment.

Olive oil is monounsaturated, so saturated fat content in the oil is nil. Monounsaturated fat decreases LDL and decreases the risk of heart disease. It's no wonder that Popeye and Bluto are always fighting over Olive Oyl.

If HDL is Cholesterol Heaven, What is Cholesterol Hell?

Any food produced from land animals, or from coconut and palm oils, is bad news, containing saturated fats. Stuff like stuffed-crust, meat-lover's pizza contains as much as 10 grams of saturated fat, which is about the same as a McDonald's Quarter Pounder.

Saturated fat raises LDL. Transfatty acids, produced by adding hydrogen molecules to vegetable oils, are solid fats which raise LDL—bad—and lower HDL—bad—(double your badness). Time to skip the pepperoni and ask for the pepperoncini!

Go Ahead, Eat Me...

Sweet potatotes: loaded with carotenoids, vitamin C, potassium and fiber.

Broccoli: power-packed with vitamin C, carotenoids and folic acid, and a proud member of the cruciferous vegetable group, which is jam-packed with anti-cancer properties.

Spinach and kale: super sources of calcium, fiber, vitamin C, and Omega-3 fatty acids.

Asparagus: not only scrumptious, it is also loyal, and odorizes your urine. Asparagus contains methionine, the same sulfur compound found in rotten eggs, onions, garlic, and in the secretions of skunks. If you don't want your urine to smell funny, pass on the asparagus; or, better yet, pass it over to me—yum.

Carbs and Carps

To carve muscles, eat carbs. When you eat carbohydrates, you maximize your stores of glycogen, which your body uses for energy (along with fat) during a workout. Pasta, rice, and white bread are rich in carbohydrates but

HDL and LDL

The higher your HDL and the lower your LDL, the younger your arteries. Think of monounsaturated fats as Liquid Plumber for the heart, keeping it unclogged. It is okay to listen to stereo, but eat mono. —

Carotenoids

What the heck are carotenoids? No, it is not putting carrots up your nose—that would be carrot-adenoids. Your body converts carotenoids into vitamin A, and A is AOK, especially when it is from a plant, not a capsule.

Carotenoids are also excellent antioxidants, which take on the ultra-dangerous free radicals. (You are on your own, however, with all the free ultra-conservatives.) —

have a high glycemic index which raises blood insulin levels rapidly, which decreases blood sugar levels and promotes hunger. High glycemic index foods also promote fat storage. 100% whole grain bread contains more vitamins and minerals than white bread, which should be consumed only in small amounts.

Along with carbs, eat an occasional carp, because fish is brain food (do fish eat brains?).

Eating fish also reduces the likelihood of heart disease, Alzheimer's, and cancer, not to mention mad cow disease. Fish such as albacore tuna and salmon contain Omega-3 fatty acids. If you are wild about salmon, make it wild salmon, not farmed, because wild has more Omega-3s.

Good Cop, Bad Cop

Watermelon good, water buffalo not good. One is a refreshingly sweet source of carotenoids; the other is simply caribou.

Orange good, orangutan not good. One has an abundance of vitamin C, and lots of folic acid, potassium, and fiber. The other is unable to manipulate its thumbs, and smells yucky.

Cantaloupe good, antelope not so good. One provides your daily requirements of vitamins A and C, in just a quarter slice. If you slice the other, it will bleed all over the home where the buffalo roam.

Beans good. Then again, beans not so good. You can't beat them as a low-cost source of low-fat protein, but it is a double-edged bean, because even though they are good for your heart, the more you eat...you know that dumb song.[2]

Carrots good, carats even better. What's up, Doc? If you eat carrots like that famous cwazy wabbit, the chances of having to see a doc is greatly reduced. Carrots provide 360% of your daily minimum requirement for beta-carotene, which means special nutrition for your eyes. You know the old joke about never seeing a rabbit wearing glasses? I have never seen one; then again, that may be because I was not wearing my glasses.

Garlic, good. You mean the stinking rose? Experiments by competent scientists, as well as incompetent Italians, have shown that regular consumption of garlic may have the following physical effects:

● lowers blood pressure

● helps reduce atherosclerotic buildup within the arterial system

● lowers or helps to regulate blood sugar

● helps prevent blood clots from forming thus reducing the possibility of strokes and thromboses

● helps prevent cancer, especially of the digestive system

Garlic also makes for a very stinking good-night kiss, unless both of you are garlic lovers.

---

[2]Other great sources of protein include non-fat cottage cheese and yogurt, white meat, and fish. Some say worms and roaches, too, but they are acquired tastes, like borscht.

Speaking of Stinking

To get your vitamins, minerals, fiber, and complex carbohydrates, and help lower your intake of fat, stock that fridge of yours with plenty of grain products, vegetables, and fruits. Keep in mind, however, that in a recent alarming poll conducted by an appliance manufacturer, it was discovered that nearly 25% of Americans clean out their refrigerators less than twice a year, rendering their fridges breeding grounds for health-threatening mold and fungus.

If your fridge smells worse than it looks, try wearing a clothespin on your nose, or put an open box of baking soda in it (in the fridge, not in your nose).

Ugh, Sweep It Under the Rug! Facts That are Hard to Swallow

A popular natural oat and honey granola with a picture of Hopalong Cassidy on the label (or is it William Penn?) contains three teaspoons of sugar per half cup, and more artery-clogging fat than even a McDonald's burger. Toss it, or turn your heart into goo.

A well-known bakery with a name like Exitmann (or is it enema man?) has a "rich frosted" donut that contains as much saturated fat as nine strips of bacon. Let's dunk the donuts and chew the fat; taste it, don't swallow it.

That "cup of noodle" brand containing pre-fried and pre-salted noodles prepared in artery-clogging palm oil has six times as much sodium as you find in potato chips. Avoid it at all costs, or get thee to a coroner.

Eating fried food is like shoving gum, or Playdough, into your aorta.

Raw spelled backwards is war. Sushi spelled backwards is ihsus.[3] And speaking of raw, ever wonder if cannibals, when they eat chicken, say it tastes like humans?

Don't Forget to Water Yourself

Eat, drink, and be hydrated. When you are thirsty, drink.

Some may recommend that you drink eight glasses of water a day. That is not necessary, unless you enjoy going to the bathroom frequently.

Cannibal Fact

Cannibal Fact of the Week: Attila the Hun was said to have eaten two of his sons. ("Man, today Dad really chewed me out!") Not only was he a lousy father, he was a lousy cook. He cooked his meat by placing it between his thighs and the hot, sweaty back of his horse. It's rare, it's raw, it's gnarly! ⸺

---

[3]Backwards spelled backwards is sdrawkcab.

Beer vs. Red Wine

Drinking beer with dinner works better than drinking red wine for controlling homocysteine, a blood factor that promotes heart disease. If you are homocysteinephobic, drink more beer. Folate also causes disintegration of homocysteine. —

A large percentage of disease in the United States may be due to improper nutrition: too much fat, too little fiber, and not enough fruits and vegetables. If you eat right and in moderation, and get exercise, you will not only ward off illness, you will have the low body fat of a lingerie model.

An Interview...

...with the 999½-Year-Old Hypochondriac[1]

He is old, really old, and doesn't look a day over 167. Here are his secrets...

Q: How about a word from a man who has been around the block approximately 364,819 times, give or take a block?

A: Back in the old days, we didn't call them blocks, we called them clans, spelled with a "c" not a "k." This was back before sheets were invented.

Q: Wow, you are 999-and-a-half-years-old!

A: Young, I am 999-and-a-half-years-young!

Q: I stand corrected.

A: Why stand when you can sit? That is one of my secrets to living a long life.

Q: Tell us, what are your other secrets?

A: To find out, it's gonna cost you, young man, plenty.

Q: Okay, how much?

A: How about an ox?

Q: That sounds doable. Okay, one ox in return for your secret.

A: Promise you won't tell Victoria? She can't keep a secret. I just peeked into one of her saucy catalogues and boy-oh-boy, if that Gutenberg kid had only known what his printing press could do, he would have invented the centerfold. Oy, I must be having a senior moment, since I forgot what we were just talking about.

Q: Your secret to long life?

A: My secret to a long life is this: stay away from fried foods.

Q: That's it?

A: That, and avoid deadly plagues.

Q: Especially black ones, I bet.

---

[1]With apologies, and heartfelt thanks, to Carl Reiner and Mel Brooks.

A: Plagues once came in only one color. Today, thanks to Henry Ford, they come in red, green, and even chartreuse.

Q: There must be other reasons why you have lived so long.

A: Yes, and it's gonna cost you another ox.

Q: Okay, shoot.

A: Bang!

Q: Shoot is just an expression that means, "Go ahead!" Tell me more.

A: Okay, three words: poisonous blow darts. Stay far away from those deadly little suckers. A poisonous blow dart will kill you faster than a plague.

Q: I will make a note of that. Fried foods, deadly plagues, poisonous blow darts—anything else?

A: I always keep an eye on my cholesterol.

Q: That makes sense, but I didn't know people were aware of cholesterol in medieval times.

A: We knew all about cholesterol, we just didn't call it that. We called it Exekiel's crud.

Q: I take it you avoided fatty foods.

A: Kept my distance, especially from that crud Exekiel was hawking. Usually, I was more than a hop, skip, and jump away.

Q: Hop, skip, and jump sounds like an ancient aerobics workout.

A: Kept the ol' ticker tocking, or the ol' tocker ticking. Before we had clocks, it kept the ol' sundial dialing. We learned this from watching animals, rabbits in particular. The rabbits hopped, I skipped, and jumped 'em. A delicious workout if you liked rabbit!

Q: Grocery stores did not come along for nearly 900 years, so one reason you have lived so long, I assume, is that you cooked your food from scratch. Right?

A: Right!

Q: And, you ate a diet of high fiber and low fat?

A: Right again.

Q: Plus fish for the brain.

A: You are a very smart young man. For strong bones, I also drank foods high in calcium, like milk (I also got sunshine to make my calcium work). Aaah, milking, that was a piece of cake. And butter! What a pain in the butt butter was!

Q: Margarine didn't come along for another nine centuries.

A: No margarine then, but we had Marge; whatta kisser.

Q: She was pretty?

A: Not this Marge. She was as ugly as a baboon, but whatta kisser! She would kiss anything, even an ox. Once she pressed her lips against an ox's mouth so long it dropped dead of suffocation. You might say she was the world's first ox murderer.

Q: You are a funny guy.

A: If Henny Youngman was around today, I would sell him that joke for a nice young rooster.

Q: Getting back to butter...

A: To get butter, it took a lot of churning, not what I do best. Someone was always giving me directions. Churn left, churn right, churn here, churn there. I was always taking the wrong churn, and ended up under the cow. That's okay, as too much butter is not good for the ol' ticker.

Q: Lots of heart disease back in the old days?

A: Well, if a ten-foot long, twelve-hundred-pound saber-tooth tiger suddenly wandered into your cave, you would have a coronary, too.[2]

Q: I suppose I would. But, look at you—you survived.

A: Before planes, trains and automobiles, we walked everywhere. On my 137th birthday, my nineteenth wife and I...

Q: Nineteen wives?

A: In fact, I married fifty times, almost as many times as Liz Taylor and Mickey Rooney combined. My nineteenth wife gave me some camels and a chariot. Boy, did I used to love smoking camels while cruising in my chariot, until I learned it was bad for my heart.

Q: Smoking?

A: No, chariots! I saw one run over my old bridge partner, Og. His name used to be Ogstein, but he changed it to avoid crucifixion. Didn't matter, though, because some reckless, drunken chariot driver ran right over him, crushing his chest flat as a pancake. Bad for the heart, chariots were.

Q: So, you have experienced adversity over the past ten centuries?

A: You said it! One day it's bubonic, the next day it's cholera, another day it's Attila the Hun—no wonder my pals from the old neighborhood are no longer still around.

Q: You managed to survive.

A: I survived because I am a hypochondriac. You name it, I worry about getting it. When you worry about getting everything, somehow you manage to avoid everything.

Q: Your secret is hypochondria?

A: Yes, hypochondria and safe sax.

Q: You mean safe sex?

A: No, safe sax. When I play a wind instrument, my lips never touch the mouthpiece. It's a haven for germs.

Q: If your lips don't touch the mouthpiece, how do you play?

---

[2]Every caveman had a health club. The moment a saber-tooth tiger tiptoed into his cave—bam! Og would club the half-ton carnivore right over his striped noggin. Back then, every caveman carried a health club.

A: Not very well, thank you.

Q: Thank you for your time.

A: Time is all I got. Take as much as you want, but it's gonna cost you.

Q: I am out of oxen.

A: In that case, I am out of time. Tootaloo!

Q: So long.

A: You should live so long!

section four

Appendices

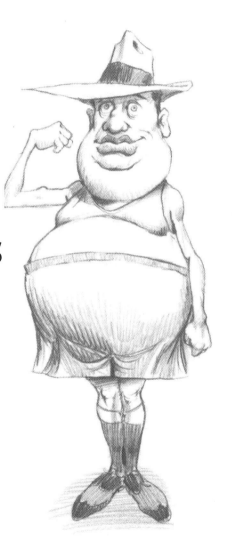

Appendix One

Quick Tips for Your Diet

WHITE LITE: avoid the skin and dark meat when you eat chicken or turkey. You'll be gobbling fat if you eat it!

GAME ON THE RANGE: wild game such as buffalo and venison is lean and less saturated with fats than veal, beef, or ham.

DAIRY DIESEL: protein contains the amino acid phenylalanine (mostly found in milk), which stimulates the production of the alertness chemicals norepinephrine, epinephrine, and dopamine.

GOOD FOR YOU? chocolate does not cause acne and it's good for you in small doses, especially dark chocolate.

FAT FILBERT: nuts such as filberts, almonds, and walnuts are high in fats, but mostly good, monounsaturated fats.

BIRD NAP: carbohydrates contain tryptophan, which stimulates the production of seratonin, and may cause drowsiness. Tryptophan is also found in turkey.

FREEZER FRESH: frozen foods are often (though not always) as nutritious as fresh, raw food.

PICK O' THE PRODUCE: especially good for you are dark greens, such as spinach and broccoli, and some red and orange foods—like tomatoes and carrots. Stay colorful!

HEAT TREAT: heating tomatoes releases more lycopene, which may help protect against prostate disorders.

BEST BUY: one cannot do better than cruciferous veggies for vitamins, minerals, and fiber content. Some examples are broccoli, cauliflower, kale, and Brussels sprouts; they are also known to help prevent cancer.

CAVEAT EMPTOR: until the regulation of herbal remedies improves, let the buyer beware!

TRANS-FAT CALCULATOR: trans-fats are in shortening, fried foods, and many margarines. Trans-fatty acids raise LDL (bad cholesterol) levels and lower HDL (good cholesterol) levels. They also raise triglyceride levels. Saturated fats such as butter raise LDLs and HDLs. To determine how much trans-fat is in your favorite snack foods, add up the listed constituent fat totals, and if they are shy of the total fat content, the difference is likely the hidden trans-fat content. New regulations are changing the way trans-fats are labeled.

CANCER FIGHTING FOODS: these include natural phytochemicals such as:

- Indoles: broccoli, cauliflower

- Hioallyl derivatives: garlic and onions kill bacteria and viruses.

- Antioxidants: carotene, vitamins C and E promote cell health.

- Phenotic compounds: fruits, vegetables, black and green tea

- Flavonoids: soy products and apples promote healthy cell growth.

THE RICE STUFF:

- Choose whole grains over highly processed flour or rice.

- Restrict white carb-rich foods including sugar, white bread, white rice, and white potatoes (these are high glycemic index foods).

- Eat high fiber fruits and veggies, such as carrots and apples.

- Add vinegar or lemon juice to carbs to lower glycemic index up to 30%.

SUGAR SCAM: scientific studies prove sugar does not make children hyperactive.

DON'T BELIEVE THE HYPE: honey and brown sugar offer no significant nutritional advantage over other sugars.

ALBACORE AND OMEGA: tuna, salmon, herring, and sardines are highest in Omega-3 fatty acids, which lower blood pressure.

SOUPED UP: liquids, especially chunky soup, may curb appetite by filling you up.

Appendix Two

Weight Training and Cardio Quick Tips

JOIN-A-GYM: 13% of Americans are members of a health facility. More people join to lift weights than to lose weight. Healthy people like to exercise more than unhealthy people; active participation does not always follow membership and turnover is high, especially as the year progresses.

TAKE A BREAK: it takes 48 hours to build new muscle after exercise breaks it down; make sure to get adequate rest after your workouts.

GO, NOT SHOW: select a trainer based on certification with the ACSM (American College of Sports Medicine) or ACE (American Council on Exercise). Identify your needs: time, place, personality, and your expectations.

ONE-MINUTE RULE: rest for one minute between sets, and for two minutes before moving on to the next exercise.

MOVE IT: lifting weights every other day is optimal: taking a walk several times a week also has significant benefits.

WEIGHT GAIN: when you can do 12 reps with good form, add pounds to your weight load.

UNDER WRAPS: long sleeves and long pants keep muscles warm, which delays fatigue.

YEARN TO BURN: the greater your muscle mass, the faster your metabolism, and vice versa. Aerobic exercise ups your metabolism and burns more calories throughout the day.

HEART HELPER: exercise raises HDL (good) cholesterol and lowers LDL (bad) cholesterol.

MUSCULAR MEMORY: muscles have memory, so if you lift weights for years, your muscles will respond better than the muscles of someone who has seldom exercised.

STRETCH DON'T STRAIN: to possibly lower your risk of injury, warm up for 3 to 5 minutes on a stationary bike, followed by slow, sustained stretching; stretch again after your workout. Keep in mind that stretched muscles are, by definition, more resilient, although injury may still occur.

DON'TS OF EXERCISE:

- Don't skip exercises.

- Don't do the same activity for prolonged periods.

- Don't maintain your activity at too rapid a pace.

- Don't ignore pain!

SAUNA STRESS: prolonged time in a sauna after your workout can cause dehydration, nausea, dizziness, and headaches, and may delay muscle recovery.

MUSCLE BLIND: weight machines work just as well as barbells and dumbbells; your muscles cannot tell the difference. Beginners should probably use machines, as they are easier to use, control form, and are less likely to cause injury.

HARDER, FASTER: it is better to increase the intensity of your workout than to increase the length of the workout.

SAVVY SCULPTING: always try to work your large muscles before refining the smaller muscles. First sculpt a basic shape, then fine-tune the details.

HALF-AND-HALF: although regular exercise can help keep weight down, you will need to burn 3,200 calories to lose a pound (running a mile burns approximately 100 calories). Diet and exercise combine to produce the most efficient weight loss.

LEAN TOWARD HEALTH: exercise can redistribute your weight from fat mass to lean mass. Excess weight in the form of fat is shown to contribute to many cancers: the leaner, the cleaner.

Appendix Three

Glossary: Diet Terms

ANTIOXIDANTS: a group of vitamins, minerals, and enzymes that protect your body from attack by free radicals, which are destructive particles that form in the body. A few antioxidants prove that Mother Nature is not just "all work and no play." Antioxidants are found in abundance in green veggies, red wine, dark chocolate, and in vitamins C and E.

CAROTENOIDS: your body converts carotenoids—specifically beta-carotene, which is found in carrots and other veggies—into vitamin A. You need this vitamin for healthy eyes, for your immune system, and to prevent skin disorders like acne. Start snacking like Bugs does! And, for you meat lovers, preformed vitamin A is found in meat and egg yolks.

DIETARY FIBER: regular ingestion of fiber lowers blood cholesterol, stabilizes blood sugar levels, and corrects disorders of the large intestine. Because fiber passes through your digestive tract relatively intact, it helps keep things functioning normally by scrubbing you from the inside out. Oat bran and wheat bran are important sources of fiber found in cereal, breads, and muffins; snack on these goodies and stay clean!

THE SKINNY ON FATS: here is a rundown on some common fats, and some advice about which to eat and which to avoid. (All fats have the same number of calories.)

MONOUNSATURATED FATS: very good for you. You can get fat if you guzzle olive oil, but it is less harmful.

PARTIALLY HYDROGENATED FATS: the worst of all fats, including vegetable shortening, found in most processed foods. These fats, which are also known as trans-fatty acids, float around in your blood stream and clog your arteries because they have an unnatural chemical structure. Just think of how long supermarket cookies and crackers last on the shelf. Partially hydrogenated fats raise triglycerides and LDLs, and they lower beneficial HDLs.

OMEGA-6: you likely get enough corn oil and soy oil in your regular diet–no need to go out of your way for these. Excessive Omega-6 intake decreases absorption of Omega-3s.

SATURATED FATS: found in perennial favorites such as butter and other dairy products (except non-fat varieties), and beef and other meats. Saturated fats are best to avoid. Processed and fast foods are also super-saturated with saturated fats. These fats make your body produce more cholesterol, which raises blood cholesterol levels, thereby increasing the risk of cardiovascular disease.

FRIED FOOD: stay away from all fried foods, if possible. Heated fat (such as in a deep fryer) develops free radicals, which are known carcinogens (cancer-producers).

INTESTINAL FLORA: friendly flora such as acidophilous and bifidus are crucial to the healthy function of your digestive tract. A loss of friendly flora can lead to overabundance of "bad" bacteria and yeasts, such as candida. Eating yogurt with live acidophilus cultures is a good way to keep things in balance.

MINERALS: several major minerals are required for health, including calcium, magnesium, zinc, selenium, chromium, boron, copper, iodine, manganese, phosphorus, sulfur, potassium, and iron (phew!). Many are

crucial for boosting your endurance when training and exercising. Luckily, most of these are supplied by your regular, healthy, balanced diet.

PHYTOCHEMICALS: found in fresh raw fruits and vegetables. Phytochemicals are associated with the prevention and/or treatment of cancer, diabetes, cardiovascular disease, and hypertension.

VEGETARIAN DIET: weight training and vegetarianism are not necessarily mutually exclusive.

VITAMINS: you may need to take daily multiple vitamins if you have unusual dietary habits. And, you have nothing to lose by taking them!

Appendix Four

Glossary: Cardio and Fitness Training

CARDIOVASCULAR EXERCISE: crucial to fitness training and general health maintenance. Cardiovascular exercise lowers cholesterol, normalizes blood sugar, and reduces hypertension, thereby reducing the risk of heart disease. Additional benefits of heart health are deep, restful sleep and enhanced mood.

PILATES: a specialized set of exercises in which you work against your own body weight to develop strength and balance with emphasis on back and abdominal strength. Physically demanding, Pilates was developed by a man who wanted to create a perfect workout for ballet dancers.

SWIMMING: benefiting upper body, mid-section, and legs all at once, swimming is a great way to improve your cardiovascular fitness. No need to fret about torn ligaments and sore knees; swimming is the most ergonomic cardio workout of all.

WALKING: walking has a relatively low injury rate. It strengthens your bones and provides aerobic benefits when you walk fast. The Surgeon General recommends 30 to 60 minutes a day of moderate walking to realize a decreased risk of heart disease, diabetes, cancer, stroke, and other maladies.

Walkers also live longer and are healthier, in general. Results from a Nurse's Health Study show significant decreases in breast cancer and Type II diabetes in women who, for two years at a time, engaged in brisk walking or other vigorous exercise for 7 hours a week, and as little as 3 hours a week for heart disease reduction. Brisk walking was defined as 3-3.9 miles per hour, or 15-20 minutes per mile.

RUNNING: among the benefits of running is weight loss and increased HDL levels (good cholesterol), according to a year-long Stanford University study. A National Runners' Health survey found that waist circumference, blood pressure, and resting heart rate are lower in male runners, as compared to those who do not engage in physical exercise.

YOGA: an ancient East Indian tradition involving the cultivation of mental and physical health, which has been modified for a western audience. The practice has a spiritual component, which is largely de-emphasized in the average gym. Yoga increases strength, flexibility, and concentration. If you have been feeling "old," yoga will help to stretch out that feeling.

Appendix Five

A Phew Rules of Gym Etiquette

RE-RACK YOUR WEIGHTS: Not only is it good etiquette, it prevents stubbed toes. It may also prevent a broken nose—yours.

QUIET PLEASE: If you are strong enough to lift the weight, you are strong enough to set it down quietly. Don't be a "crank and banger."

PICK UP AFTER YOURSELF: Wipe down the sink after use; toss towels into the hampers. And remember not to leave your bottles lying around.

PHONE LATER: Keep your cell phone the heck out of the gym.

ELBOW ROOM: Give others the right of way, and plenty of space during their bench-pressing, stair-stepping, weight lifting, and other activities.

GIVE IT UP: Allow others to work with the equipment between your sets, especially if you are sitting around, socializing, or ogling your reflection.

LEAN AND CLEAN: Use a dry towel to wipe down sweat-soaked machines after your use.

GRIP IT: Do not spit on the handlebars to get a good grip. Some irked jerk may get a good grip...around your neck.

DRESS: Attire yourself adequately and appropriately.

TATTOOS: Observe and respect.

NOISE/SOUNDS: These are not necessary while training.

SHARE, ENCOURAGE, AND BE ENTHUSIASTIC!

Keep It Up

Keep it up, whether at work or at play;
working out lightens and improves your day.

Living it up boosts your output and fun,
whether you are on a walk or on the run.

If you pull down a statue, it may assist a cause;
if you pull a hamstring, your endeavors will pause.

Good luck, best wishes, now get out and go!
since Don and Harry have finished their show.

If you are tired, elated, sweaty,
and all done with procrastination,
I have succeeded in providing a fun
and productive education!

—D.L.

Final Words from the Author

Actually, the last page!

- Gymnasium "mental intensity" is important.

- After all, gym-going or going to the gym is similar to a religion.

  1. Regular attendance

  2. Ritual orientation

  3. Guilt/atonement

  4. Sacerdotal instruction

- No animals were harmed in the making of this book, although a lot of brave carrots fell in the line of duty.

- Recently, I had a mole removed. The doctor said, "On a scale of 1 to 10, it's benign."

- Older today than yesterday, I am younger than I will be tomorrow.

- Then again, if I eat right and exercise regularly, I may be younger tomorrow than I am today.

- Life begins at 80, especially if you just completed a 50-year prison sentence.

- At your gym, you may be wondering about all the pickup trucks—why so many? Do health nuts drive trucks? Or, are truckers just health nuts?

- Whatever you need, from a building contractor to a plumber or an electrician, just go to your gym's parking lot.

- If you worked out in formal attire, would you call your gym James?

- If birthdays are dumb, I look forward to getting dumb and dumber.

- Remember to breathe in, breathe out.

- He who laughs last is the last one to get the joke.

- So, keep it up, upper, uppest—forever!

  —D.L.